LTH LAW

FOR NURSES

mond

.D, DSA, AHSM

er at Law and Emeritus Professor of the University of Glamorgan

Frances H. Barker

MA (Oxon), MIInfSci, AIL

Blackwell

Science

Blackwell Science Ltd, a Blackwell Publishing company
Editorial offices:
Blackwell Science Ltd, 9600 Garsington Road, Oxford OX4 2DQ, UK
    Tel: +44 (0) 1865 776868
Blackwell Publishing Inc., 350 Main Street, Malden, MA 02148-5020, USA
    Tel: +1 781 388 8250
Blackwell Science Asia Pty Ltd, 550 Swanston Street, Carlton, Victoria 3053, Australia
    Tel: +61 (0)3 8359 1011

First published 1996
Reprinted 1998, 1999, 2001, 2003, 2005

Library of Congress Cataloging-in-Publication Data is available

ISBN-10: 0-632-03989-2
ISBN-13: 978-0632-03989-0

A catalogue record for this title is available from the British Library

Set in 10/13pt Melior
by DP Photosetting, Aylesbury, Bucks
Printed and bound by Replika Press Pvt. Ltd., India

The publisher's policy is to use permanent paper from mills that operate a sustainable forestry policy, and which has been manufactured from pulp processed using acid-free and elementary chlorine-free practices. Furthermore, the publisher ensures that the text paper and cover board used have met acceptable environmental accreditation standards.

For further information on Blackwell Publishing, visit our website:
www.blackwellpublishing.com

Contents

Foreword		*v*
Abbreviations used in this book		*vi*
Acknowledgements		*vi*
1	Introduction	1
2	The Code of Practice and other guidance	6
3	Definitions of mental disorder and medical recommendations for admission	12
4	Admission to hospital under Part II of the Act	20
5	Admission to hospital under Part III of the Act: mentally disordered offenders	33
6	Provision of information to the patient and nearest relative	45
7	The nearest relative	52
8	Consent to treatment	59
9	Appeals against detention	72
10	Leave with consent under section 17	82
11	Returning the patient to hospital	86
12	Entering premises to take a mentally disordered person	92
13	Police powers of arrest and place of safety	95
14	Transfer of patients	100
15	Guardianship	105
16	The role of the approved social worker and the social worker	110
17	Community care	115
18	Rectification of documents	121
19	The mental health managers	129
20	The Mental Health Act Commission	133
21	Offences under the Act and staff protection against court action by the patient	139
22	Conclusion	148
Glossary		150
Table of Cases		154
Table of Statutes and Statutory Instruments		155
Appendix I(A) Extracts from the Mental Health Act 1983		157

Appendix I(B)   Extracts from the Mental Health
(Patients in the Community) Act 1995   168
Appendix I(C)   Code of Practice (section 118) –
Procedures to be set up as detailed in
the Code   173
Appendix I(D)   Law Commission Report No. 231,
Mental Incapacity 1995 HMSO   175
Appendix II   Forms and leaflets with examples of
non-statutory forms   176
Example A: MHA 1983 Leaflet 1   179
Example B: Patients Rights –
Proforma for informing   181
Example C: Mental Health Act 1983 –
section 62   182
Example D: MHRT 1   183
Example E: MHRT 2   185
Example F: Form for recording section
17 leave   187
Example G: Application for admission
to a place of safety   188
Example H: Implementing section 17
after-care   189
Example J: MHAC visit announcement   193
Useful Addresses   194
Bibliography   197
Index   199

Foreword

Nurses are involved in the delivery of humane and high quality care to their patients. Nowhere are these objectives more important than in the field of mental health, and one important quality standard to be applied to the work of a nurse is that it is lawful.

This book sets out with great clarity the legal framework provided by the Mental Health Act and examines in helpful detail those parts of the legislation that are particularly relevant. It will make an important contribution to the maintenance of the highest standards in psychiatric and mental health nursing.

William Bingley
Chief Executive Officer
Mental Health Act Commission

Abbreviations used in this book

ACAS	Advisory, Conciliation and Arbitration Service
DHA	District Health Authority
DHSS	Department of Health and Social Security
DoH	Department of Health
ECT	Electro-convulsive Therapy
FHSA	Family Health Services Authority
HA	Health Authority
HC	Health Circular
HMSO	Her Majesty's Stationery Office
HSC	Health Services Commission
MHAC	Mental Health Act Commission
MHRT	Mental Health Review Tribunal
NHSME	National Health Service Management Executive
PRN	Pro re nata (see Glossary)
RMO	Responsible Medical Officer
SI	Statutory Instrument (see Glossary)
SOAD	Second Opinion Appointed Doctor
UKCC	United Kingdom Central Council for Nursing, Midwifery and Health Visiting

Acknowledgements

Grateful thanks are due to Eric Chitty who commented on the very first draft, and to Monty Graham and William Bingley who have commented on this final version.

We acknowledge the copyright of HMSO for extracts and forms from statutes and statutory instruments, and thank Powys Health Care Trust and Rosemary Goode, Medical Records Officer, for permission to use their forms.

Chapter 1   Introduction

Compulsory care and treatment of mentally ill people in the UK is governed essentially by the Mental Health Act 1983 (hereafter referred to as 'the Act') and the Code of Practice (prepared under section 118) first published in 1990 and reviewed periodically by the Secretary of State. A second edition was published in 1993.

The aim of this book is to provide an introduction and practical guide to the law and directives embodied in the Act and Code. It should be of value to those who are undergoing their initial training as registered nurses. It should also be of assistance to all nurse practitioners, whether or not they intend to seek registration status for nursing the mentally ill or the mentally impaired. Any nurse in any specialty may find that her patients are suffering from mental disorder and she should have an understanding of the legal principles and a book for easy referral.

The book is also designed for the nurse trained in the care of the mentally ill or mentally handicapped who, although she might once have worked in a large psychiatric ward with regular admissions under mental health legislation, now finds herself working in a small community home for the mentally disordered where admissions under the Act might occur at a rate of less than one a year. In such circumstances it is easy for knowledge of the legal processes to become rusty and it is essential to have an easy reference book covering the basic procedures.

It is also recognized that by far the majority of patients do not come under the provisions of the Act and have **informal status** (see Figure 1.1). In each chapter therefore, where relevant, part of the chapter concentrates on the legal issues which concern the care of the informal patient.

On the difficult issue of gender specific terminology, we have often referred to a nurse as 'she', but this is simply for convenience and to avoid clumsy usages. There is, of course, a much higher proportion of male nurses in mental health nursing than in other areas of the profession.

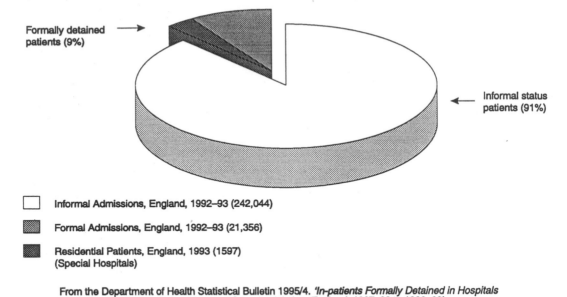

Formally detained
patients (9%)

Informal status
patients (91%)

☐ Informal Admissions, England, 1992–93 (242,044)

▨ Formal Admissions, England, 1992–93 (21,356)

▮ Residential Patients, England, 1993 (1597)
(Special Hospitals)

From the Department of Health Statistical Bulletin 1995/4. *'In-patients Formally Detained in Hospitals Under the Mental Health Act 1993 and Other Legislation, England: 1987–88 to 1992–93'.*

Figure 1.1   Mental disorder – hospital admissions (England).

It is hoped that the book may also be useful to those working in other disciplines, such as occupational therapists, physiotherapists, psychologists and others, who might have occasional contact with the statutory procedures and need to refresh their memory.

Some facts and figures

The purpose of the Act is to set out the law. Those working in the mental health area must be aware of the law in order to make valid decisions as to whether a person's condition is serious enough to warrant loss of liberty and/or compulsory treatment, and what procedures should be followed. The powers of the Act should be invoked only when really necessary.

The number of formal admissions in England in 1992–93 was 21 356. This is 44 detained patients in every 100 000 of population. The number of residential patients in the Special Hospitals in 1993 was 1597. Detained patients represent about 10% of those in hospital for mental disorder; the majority are 'informal status' patients. The number of informal admissions in England in 1992–93 was 242 044 (see Figure 1.1). These figures are from the Department of Health Statistical Bulletin No. 1995/4, *In-*

Patients Formally Detained in Hospital Under The Mental Health Act 1983 and Other Legislation.

An overview of admission to psychiatric hospitals

For clarification it should be explained that there are four distinct forms of admission:

- informal admission,
- civil admission under compulsion,
- compulsory admission from the criminal courts, and
- compulsory transfers from prison to hospital.

Informal admission

The vast majority of patients are admitted informally, i.e. without any formality or statutory procedures. Section 131 covers this situation and is discussed in Chapter 4. The Act does not cover such patients, except where brain surgery for mental disorder or hormonal implants to reduce sexual drive in men are being contemplated and then section 57 applies (see Chapter 8).

Civil admission under compulsion

This is covered under Part II of the Act and is discussed in Chapters 3, 4, 12, 13 and 15.

Compulsory admission from the courts compulsory transfers from prison

These are both considered in Chapter 5 and are covered in Part III of the Act.

Structure of the Mental Health Act 1983

The Mental Health Act 1983 has ten parts which are as follows:

Part I   Application of the Act (including definition of mental disorder – see Chapter 3)

Part II   Compulsory Admission to Hospital and Guardianship (see Chapters 4 and 15)

Part III   Patients concerned in Criminal Proceedings or under Sentence (see Chapter 5)

Part IV   Consent to Treatment (see Chapter 8)

Part V   Mental Health Review Tribunals (see Chapter 9)

Part VI   Removal and Return of Patients within United Kingdom, etc. (not covered in this book)

Part VII   Management of Property and Affairs of Patients
            (not covered in this book)
Part VIII   Miscellaneous Functions of Local Authorities and
            the Secretary of State (see Chapters 16, 17 and 20)
Part IX   Offences (see Chapter 21)
Part X   Miscellaneous and supplementary (see Chapters 6,
            12 and 19)

How does the Act affect the detained patient?

(1)   It enables patients to be admitted specifying the grounds, the
       applicants, the procedure to be followed and the documentation
       which must be used. It also enables a detained patient who is
       absent without leave to be compulsorily returned.

(2)   It regulates the care of the patient during the detention by laying
       down rules in relation to the giving of treatment, the information
       to be provided, the right of access to the Mental Health Act
       Commission, and leave of absence and recall.

(3)   It enables a patient to obtain discharge from the section through
       a nearest relative, or by application to the Hospital Manager
       and/or Mental Health Review Tribunal, or by the Responsible
       Medical Officer.

(4)   It requires provision to be made for the after-care of patients
       detained under certain specified sections.

       The after-care provisions were strengthened and supple-
    mented in the 1995 amending legislation and the relevant sec-
    tions are shown in Appendix I(B).

Layout of this book

In some ways the Act of 1983 belongs to another era. Even
though the move to community care had been professed as
essential for many years, real progress in closing or cutting
down the bed numbers of the old institutions has only been
effective in recent times. The 1983 Act is essentially concerned
with admission into an institution. There is no provision for a
community treatment order and the guardianship sections (see
Chapter 14) have been used erratically across the country, with
some social services authorities/departments making very little
use of them. However it is recognized that far fewer seriously
mentally disordered patients are now living in an institution

and the book therefore devotes some attention to the problems which arise in the care of those patients in the community.

Reference to and understanding of the actual wording of the Act is most important. Where appropriate, the relevant sections of the Act have been set out in full in Appendix I(A). For ease of reference, procedures and statutory preconditions have been shown in the form of figures, and here, to assist in understanding, minor changes to the wording have been made. It is assumed that most readers will have access to a copy of the Code of Practice (available from Her Majesty's Stationery Office (HMSO)). This is essential in order to maintain and develop good practice and in addition there is the helpful Memorandum prepared by the Department of Health and Social Services, *The Mental Health Act*. For those who have acquired a good understanding of the Act, there is the *Manual* prepared by Richard Jones which gives a full explanation of each section and the cases decided by the courts. The use which can be made of these publications is discussed in the next chapter.

Statutory documents are very important and must be completed fully and accurately. Appendix II lists the important statutory forms and gives examples of some useful non-statutory ones.

Finally it is recognized that this book should be useful as a teaching resource and therefore where appropriate exercises and questions have been set to enable tutors to take the debate and discussion further. It is for this reason that a comprehensive bibliography has also been included to enable the practitioner to follow up areas of interest.

Questions and exercises

(1) Find out where you can most easily consult the Code of Practice.

(2) Use the Code of Practice to find guidelines on the management of patients presenting special difficulties and the use of restraint and seclusion.

Chapter 2 The Code of Practice and other guidance

The Code of Practice (see section 118 of the Mental Health Act) is designed to guide nurses, registered medical practitioners, managers and other staff of hospitals and mental nursing homes and approved social workers in relation to the **admission** of patients under the Act; and also for the guidance of registered medical practitioners, nurses and members of other professions in relation to the **medical treatment** of patients suffering from mental disorder. Whilst it is therefore principally concerned with the detained patient, some of the guidance does extend to the informal patient.

Status of the Code

The Code of Practice does not have force of law, but failure to follow the Code could be referred to in evidence in legal proceedings. In this sense it is comparable with the Highway Code or the ACAS Codes on employment practices. There are good reasons for keeping to the Code unless following its provisions would be to the detriment of the patient.

Review of the Code

The Secretary of State has a statutory duty to review the Code and has delegated the monitoring of it to the Mental Health Act Commission. A consultation document had been published by the Department of Health (DoH) and a revised edition was put before Parliament in May 1993 and has been in force since November 1993. This process is on-going and an opportunity is therefore available to all those involved with the care of the mentally disordered to make suggestions for inclusions or amendments. This includes nursing staff who through their regular contact with the patients may come across anomalies or omissions in the Code.

The nurse should therefore make every effort to understand the Code and discuss the provisions. Where she feels that there are gaps or ambiguities she should make her views known to senior officers for these views to be conveyed to the Mental Health Act Commission, or be prepared to communicate with the Commission herself. She should remember that the Code should be a developing document and cover current concerns in the care of the patient.

Ways in which the Code can be of assistance

Below is a list of areas where knowledge of the contents of the Code can be used to good effect. It can be used to:

- raise standards,
- attract resources,
- clarify responsibilities,
- agree procedures, guidelines and practices,
- increase and improve level of training,
- set objectives,
- monitor and evaluate,
- prevent or end disputes between professions,
- heighten awareness of patients' rights,
- encourage multi-disciplinary work,
- encourage multi-organizational work,
- draw up check-lists, and
- press for reforms:
    - (a) internally
    - (b) at the Department of Health/Welsh Office, or
    - (d) in the professions.

It can also be:

- put in conjunction with other codes e.g. UKCC or ACAS,
- used to identify deficiencies, malpractice, weaknesses etc.,
- used to familiarize practitioners with statutory duties, and
- included in purchasing/provider agreements.

Some examples of practical use of the Code are suggested below.

(1) Take a specific aspect each week. Discuss at handover and check whether ward practice is in accordance with the guideline.

(2) Set up seminars on specific topics.

(3) Request specific sessions from the training department.

(4) Use the Code for monitoring individual multi-disciplinary practice, e.g. use of section 117.

Procedures recommended by the Code

One of the main functions of the Code is to recommend that procedures should be drawn up (usually on a multi-disciplinary basis) for a wide variety of issues. The main issues covered by the Code are listed in Figure 2.1.

Appendix I(C) lists the procedures which the Code of Practice recommends should be drawn up and the authority responsible. Many of these procedures would be prepared jointly by the local social services authority and the health service body (whether purchaser or provider). Health Authority managers include NHS trust managers where trusts have been set up. Many NHS agreements for mental health services specify the duties which providers are expected to meet under the mental health legislation.

Nurses should take steps to ensure that the relevant procedures are available in their workplace. However it cannot be assumed that once these are prepared the work is over since each procedure must be regularly reviewed and its use monitored.

Principles of the Code

The introduction to the Code sets out broad principles which should be followed in the application of the Act. These are:

- consideration of the individual,
- attention to needs,
- use of the minimum restriction necessary,
- promotion of autonomy, and
- discharge from section (legal detention) as soon as possible in the best interests of the patient.

The nurse should see the Code as a working document and remember that whilst it is written as guidance in the care of the detained patient it is also relevant to the care of the informal patient.

Other guidance

In addition to the Code of Practice the nurse should be able to refer to the Memorandum prepared by the Department of Health and Social Services in 1983. This document clarifies the text of the Act. However it does not have legal standing and if there is a

Assessment prior to possible admission under the Mental Health Act
Assessment
Part III of the Act – patients concerned with criminal proceedings
Private practice and the provisions of medical recommendations

Admission under the Mental Health Act (to hospital)
Section 2 or 3
Admission for assessment in an emergency (section 4)
Part III of the Act – patients concerned with criminal proceedings
Doctor's holding power (section 5(2))
Nurse's holding power (section 5(4))
The police power to remove to a place of safety (section 136)
Conveying to hospital
Receipt and scrutiny of documents

Admission under the Mental Health Act (to guardianship)
Guardianship (section 7)

Treatment and care in hospital
Information
Medical treatment
Medical treatment and second opinions
Part III of the Act – patients concerned with criminal proceedings
Patients presenting particular management problems
Psychological treatments
Leave of absence (section 17)
Absence without leave (section 18)
Manager's duty to review detention (section 23)
Complaints
Duties of the hospital manager
Personal searches
Visiting patients detained in hospital or a Registered Mental Nursing Home

Leaving hospital
After-care
Part III of the Act – patients concerned with criminal proceedings

Particular groups of patients
People with learning disabilities (mental handicap)
Children and young people under the age of 18

Figure 2.1   Contents of the Code of Practice – Mental Health Act 1983.

conflict between the actual provisions of the Act and the Memorandum, the former would prevail. With this in mind the nurse should nevertheless find that the Memorandum is a useful reference document.

The Mental Health Act Commission has issued leaflets giving guidance on areas which are causing confusion and need clarification. Guidance is issued in the form of Practice Notes. Practice Notes covering the administration of clozapine, the administration of medicine, and section 5(2) of the Act have been issued. They are included in the *Mental Health Act Manual* prepared by Richard Jones (see below) but copies of the Practice Notes should be widely distributed as soon as they are published.

Another useful tool to understanding the legal provisions is the *Mental Health Act Manual* written by Richard Jones. This provides a commentary on each section and includes the statutory instruments as appendices, including the Code of Practice. Once the nurse has a command of the basic provisions she should be able to use this book as a reference source.

In addition there are guides produced by MIND (National Association for Mental Health) and other groups, listed under Useful Addresses, many of which will be of use to the nurse.

The law is not static. Cases are heard where different sections of the Act and the common law powers are discussed. The most

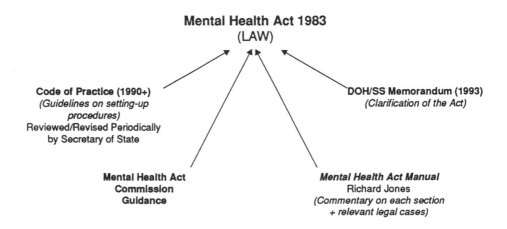

For other guides, see Bibliography

Figure 2.2   Major sources of information on mental health law.

recent edition of the *Manual* by Richard Jones will include reference to these, but the nurse should keep alert to recent cases heard since the latest edition.

Figure 2.2 summarizes the major sources of information on mental health law.

Questions and exercises

(1) Study the list of possible uses of the Code given in this chapter. Which seem most relevant to your situation? Keep a record of other uses you could make of the Code which are not cited in this book.

(2) How could you make use of the Code as a training aid and as a working document?

(3) You are aware that your hospital does not have a seclusion room; patients are being locked up in side rooms and no records are kept. Is this contrary to the Code? If so, what action would you take?

(4) You consider that one of the sections in the Code does not completely cover a situation you have encountered. What action would you take?

Chapter 3　Definitions of mental disorder and medical recommendations for admission

Mental disorder is a common condition and is suffered by a significant proportion of the population. However very few sufferers are admitted to hospital. Even so, more beds are devoted to the care of the mentally disordered than to any other specialty (admissions 44 per 100 000 population, England, 1992–93)(DoH Statistical Bulletin, NA 1995/4). Of those who receive in-patient care, 90–95% are informal patients (i.e. not compulsorily detained); only 5–10% are under compulsory detention (See Figure 1.1).

No-one can be compulsorily detained unless the statutory requirements are satisfied. An application has to be made and, unless it is an emergency situation, two doctors have to agree on the diagnosis and that the condition justifies compulsory admission. Factors involved in recommendations for admission are summarized in Figure 3.1. Much of this chapter covers the

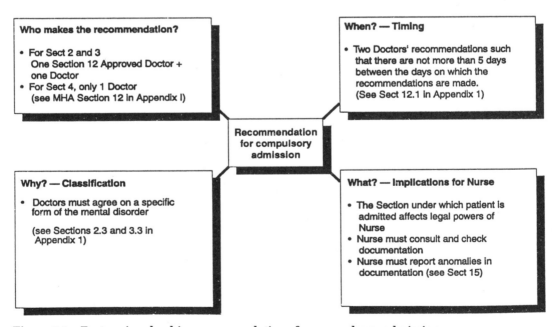

Figure 3.1　Factors involved in recommendations for compulsory admission.

definitions of mental disorder and the detailed rules under which doctors make recommendations for compulsory admission. The implications for nurses are then outlined.

Definitions

Statutory definition of 'mental disorder'

The definition of 'mental disorder' from the Mental Health Act section 1(2) is:

> 'mental illness, arrested or incomplete development of mind, psychopathic disorder and any other disorder or disability of mind and "mentally disordered" shall be construed accordingly...'

Mental illness is not further defined nor is the phrase 'any other disorder or disability of mind', but other phrases are given further definition in section 1(2):

> ' "severe mental impairment" means a state of arrested or incomplete development of mind which includes severe impairment of intelligence and social functioning and is associated with abnormally aggressive or seriously irresponsible conduct on the part of the person concerned and "severely mentally impaired" shall be construed accordingly;

> "mental impairment" means a state of arrested or incomplete development of mind (not amounting to severe mental impairment) which includes significant impairment of intelligence and social functioning and is associated with abnormally aggressive or seriously irresponsible conduct on the part of the person concerned and "mentally impaired" shall be construed accordingly;

> "psychopathic disorder" means a persistent disorder or disability of mind (whether or not including significant impairment of intelligence) which results in abnormally aggressive or seriously irresponsible conduct on the part of the person concerned...'

Even though the phrase 'mental illness' has not been defined in the Act, it has been necessary for a working definition to be used by the courts in those cases where the existence of mental disorder has been disputed. In one case (*W* v. *L* (1974)) the Court of Appeal stated that the words 'mental illness' should be regarded as ordinary words of the English language and be interpreted in the way that ordinary sensible people would interpret them. The DHSS's Memorandum does however provide examples of the symptoms which would be included in mental illness.

Guidelines in symptoms

The DHSS guidelines to mental illness symptoms are that mental illness means having an illness with one or more of the following characteristics:

● More than temporary impairment of intellectual functions shown by a failure of memory, orientation, comprehension and learning capacity;

● More than temporary alteration of mood of such degree as to give rise to the patient having a delusional appraisal of his situation, his past or his future, or that of others or to the lack of any appraisal;

● Delusional beliefs, persecutory, jealous or grandiose;

● Abnormal perceptions associated with delusional mis-interpretation of events;

● Thinking so disordered as to prevent the patient making a reasonable appraisal of his situation or having reasonable communication with others.

The mental illness should be of a nature or degree which warrants the detention of the patient in the interest of his health or safety or for the protection of others.

Statutory exclusions

The Act excludes promiscuity or other immoral conduct, sexual deviancy or dependence on alcohol or drugs from being in themselves evidence of mental disorder. The exact wording of this exclusion is given in Appendix I(A), section 1(3).

Medical recommendations for compulsory admission

Who can make medical recommendations?

At least one of the doctors making the medical recommendation must be approved for such purposes by the Secretary of State as having special experience in the diagnosis or treatment of mental disorder (section 12(2) of the Act). Regional Health Authorities were abolished in 1995 and replaced by regional branches of the NHS Management Executive. The lists of approved doctors are kept by these regional branches and such doctors are known colloquially as 'section 12 approved doctors'.

If the section 12 approved doctor does not have previous acquaintance with the patient, then section 12(2) requires that the other doctor giving the recommendation should have this. However this requirement is qualified by the words 'if practicable'. If neither of the doctors has previous acquaintance with the patient, the approved social worker or nearest relative completing the application form has to explain why. Reasons such as 'patient's usual doctor being away' may sometimes be given on the form. If possible, the responsible doctor should get in touch with the patient's doctor by telephone.

The Act attempts to maintain the **independence** of the two doctors. Where the admission is to a mental nursing home or the patient is a private patient then neither recommendation can come from doctors on the staff of the nursing home or the hospital. Where the admission is to an NHS hospital, only one of the doctors may be on the staff of that hospital. However an exception can be made under certain circumstances (see Appendix I(A), section 12(4)).

In order to ensure that the recommendations for admission are independent, many persons are prohibited from giving medical recommendations. These are in brief

- the applicant,
- partners or employees of the applicant,
- those who stand to gain from maintenance of the patient, and
- relatives of the patient or applicant.

The exact wording of section 12(5) is given in Appendix I(A). A general practitioner who is employed part-time in a hospital shall not for the purposes of section 12(5) be regarded as a practitioner on the staff (section 12(6)).

Timings for the medical recommendations

Unless the two doctors see the patient together (in which case they should complete Forms 3 or 10 for a joint medical recommendation) not more than five days must have elapsed between the days on which the separate examinations took place (section 12(1)). If, for example, one examination took place on the 8th of the month the other examination would have to be at the earliest on the 2nd or at the latest on the 14th of the same month. The medical recommendations must be signed on or before the date of the application for admission since the application must be based upon those recommendations.

Implications from the above definitions, exclusions and requirements for admission

Validity of admission to or holding in hospital

Leaving an addiction unit

In hospitals which run an addiction unit patients who wish to leave before the course has been completed cannot be compulsorily detained under the Act unless evidence of mental disorder other than their addiction is shown.

Statutory requirements

Mental disorder is not in itself sufficient to detain a person compulsorily. There must be evidence of other facts which are set out in Chapter 4 which covers admission under Part II of the Act.

Long-term sections

Different circumstances will dictate different sections of the Act under which patients are compulsorily admitted. For the longer periods of detention and guardianship it is necessary for both medical recommendations to agree on at least one specific form of mental disorder (in addition to the other requirements) for the person to be validly detained.

Patients with learning disabilities

The definition of mental disorder includes 'arrested or incomplete development of mind'. Where mental disorder rather than a specific form needs to be established, as in the short term sections (sections 2, 4, 5(2), 5(4), 135 and 136), it is not necessary to show abnormally aggressive or seriously irresponsible conduct. This means that mentally handicapped patients (now known as those with learning disabilities) come within the compulsory provisions of the Act. This has caused considerable concern to those representing this group. In practice very few of the compulsorily detained patients have learning disabilities and as appropriate facilities are provided for them in the community it is hoped that the numbers will further decline.

Discharge from section

Since the existence of mental disorder is an essential element of any compulsory admission, if that mental disorder ceases to exist the patient should be discharged from the section (i.e. no longer be compulsorily detained). **This does not necessarily mean discharge from the hospital.** There are exceptions to this in relation to restricted patients (see Chapter 5).

Validity of documents

By the time the patient is admitted there should have been a close scrutiny of the documents. Where applications are made by approved social workers, they should have confirmed that the medical recommendations are in order and appropriate for the section under which the patients have been detained. In addition there should be scrutiny of the documentation by the managers (defined in Chapter 19 and Glossary). This might include a medical scrutiny by another doctor not involved in the admission. However in spite of these checks it is still possible for the nurse to discover that the medical recommendations are not valid and she would then have a responsibility to challenge the legality of the admission.

Rectification of documents relating to medical recommendations

If errors are found in the documentation, rectification can occur in certain cases (see Chapter 18). Section 15(2) allows for rectification where one of the medical recommendations is found to be insufficient (see Appendix I(A), section 15(2)). There can be no rectification where the two medical recommendations do not refer to the same specific form of mental disorder. Nor can there be rectification outside the 14 day time limit. In such cases a fresh application must be made. In the meantime the patient would be illegally detained. Rectification on grounds other than medical recommendations is covered in Chapter 18 (Rectification of documents).

Reclassification of patients

Where it appears that a patient detained for treatment under section 3 or under a guardianship order has been wrongly diagnosed as regards mental disorder, or the diagnosis has changed, the Act allows reclassification (see Appendix I(A), section 16(1)). Section 72(5) gives a similar power to a Mental Health Review Tribunal. These sections for reclassification cannot be used to rectify documents where the two medical recommendations do not agree regarding the specific form of mental disorder. **In this case the patient would have to be reassessed.**

The informal patient

A person who is admitted to hospital without the formalities of the Act or comparable legislation is known as an 'informal' patient.

The emphasis in the Act is on treating informally wherever possible: in fact 90% of patients with mental problems are informal (see Figure 1.1). The preference is **not** to admit to hospital but to give care in the community. If it is necessary to admit, then informal admission is preferred.

Most informal patients are not governed in any way by the provisions of the Act. However those being treated for a mental disorder as defined in the Act (see Chapter 3) can be subject to the Nurse's Holding Power (section 5(4)).

If patients being treated for a mental condition outside the definition of mental disorder in the Act, for alcohol or drug abuse or for any other condition, become extremely disturbed or aggressive, the prescribed nurse cannot use the holding power. The ultimate option is compulsory admission under a section of the Act if the statutory requirements are met.

Questions and exercises

(1) Consider the following reasons given in medical recommendations for compulsory admission and state whether they would be acceptable. If not, give reasons.

'X needs treatment for alcoholism and will not come in voluntarily.'

'Z is depressed and will not eat and is not taking proper care of herself.'

'T is cantankerous with the neighbours and upsets their children.'

(2) What action would you take if you formed the view that one of the medical recommendations was inadequate?

(3) You notice that one doctor had seen the patient on 1 June and the other saw the patient on 7 June. Both recommend admission under section 2. Do these timings satisfy the statutory requirements for the purposes of compulsory admission?

(4) The Responsible Medical Officer decides that a patient detained under section 3 is not suffering from schizophrenia, but is probably suffering from a psychopathic disorder, what action should now be taken?

(5) An informal patient being treated as an in-patient in the addiction unit becomes very abusive when reprimanded for bringing

bottles of alcohol into the unit. You are not aware that she is suffering from any form of mental disorder, What action would you take if she wishes to leave? (See also Chapter 4.)

Chapter 4 Admission to hospital under Part II of the Act

Patients with a mental disorder have the same legal rights of freedom of movement as other patients unless their condition becomes such that they need to be restrained under a section of the Mental Health Act. The person considered in need of restraint may be in the community, in a non-psychiatric hospital or in a psychiatric hospital with informal status. The route of admission is dictated by the circumstances. The Act caters in the first instance for a person in the community being considered in need of assessment of their mental condition. Section 2 of the Act enables an approved social worker or nearest relative to make an application for admission for assessment. Section 3 caters for an application to be made for admission for treatment. Other sections may be used where emergency conditions exist or where the patient is already in hospital. Once a patient has been admitted under a section, his treatment for mental disorder is governed by the Act. Information about the different sections of the Act under which patients may be detained is given in this chapter. Reference should also be made to Chapters 2 and 3 of the Code of Practice.

The Act is concerned with compulsorily detained patients, but the underlying philosophy is that if admission is necessary it will be on an informal basis wherever possible. Informal status is therefore discussed under Part (1) below. Where there is an application for **compulsory** admission, the application and the medical recommendations have to state why informal admission is not appropriate. Sometimes this might be because of an absence of alternative facilities in the community and if so this has to be stated. Compulsory admission is discussed under Part (2) below. Part (3) discusses points of particular importance to the nurse in relation to compulsory detention (duration of the sections, treatment, informing the patient and nearest relative). Part (4) deals with the special case of the Nurse's Holding Power. Part (5) discusses the renewal of Section 3 (admission for treatment).

(1) Informal admission

Section 131

Very few patients suffering from mental disorder are compulsorily admitted – less than 10%. Section 131 of the Act emphasizes the freedom for patients to be admitted without formalities (see Appendix I(A), section 131(1)). Section 131 also allows for a patient to remain in hospital after he has ceased to be detained. This is important since there is a misunderstanding that ceasing to be detained means discharge from the hospital. It means discharge from the section, i.e. release from compulsory detention. Any letter notifying a detained patient that the compulsory detention has ceased should emphasize two things:

- that the patient is free to leave should he wish to do so (although, if this is contrary to medical advice, this should also be pointed out); and

- that the patient is not necessarily discharged from the hospital, but can stay there if he so wishes.

Informal patients should never be described as 'section 131 patients' since this usually implies that they have been under some form of control.

Passive patients

Informal admission does not necessarily mean voluntary admission. There are many patients who lack the capacity to consent but who do not object to being admitted to hospital for care and treatment. They are therefore admitted without any order for detention. Treatment is given to them in their best interests. (This is further discussed in Chapter 8). However, if at any stage they refuse to take treatment or wish to discharge themselves and the requirements of the Act for compulsory admission are satisfied, then an application for an order for detention could be made.

Many are concerned about this large group of patients who lack the capacity to give a valid consent and are in hospital neither by their agreement nor under a section. They are effectively outside the protection of the Act. The Law Commission has been looking at the problem relating to decision making by the mentally incapacitated adult (Report No. 119 (1991)). At present in this country there is no system for proxy decision making (Reports No. 128, No. 129 and No. 130 (1993)). The Law Commission has made a firm proposal with draft legislation (Report No. 231 (1995)) but this is a long way from being implemented (see Appendix I(D)). Clearly the nurse has an important role in protecting the interests of these passive patients. She must ensure that their best interests are always safeguarded and if at any stage she feels that the patient should be detained under a section she should bring this to the attention of the Responsible Medical Officer (RMO), the approved social worker and her senior managers.

Minors may sometimes be admitted informally, but against their will. In the case of *R* v. *Kirklees Metropolitan Borough Council, ex parte C* (1993) the Court of Appeal held that consent could be given by a parent or guardian for the admission of a minor, even when the minor herself did not wish to be admitted (section 131 discussed). This can create a grey area for staff, since, although such patients are on the one hand informal in that they are not detained under the Act, on the other hand their freedom to leave or refuse treatment is restricted.

(2) Compulsory admission (excluding mentally disordered offenders)

The Act has three sections and two sub-sections under which patients with mental disorders (other than those coming through the courts or from prison) may be compulsorily detained. These are:

Section 2	–	dealing with admission for assessment
Section 3	–	dealing with admission for treatment
Section 4	–	dealing with emergency admission for assessment
Section 5(2)	–	dealing with detention of patients already in hospital
Section 5(4)	–	dealing with emergency restraint by nurses of informal in-patients being treated for mental disorder (Nurse's Holding Power).

These sections are outlined below. Important areas in which they differ are summarized in Figure 4.1. These are:

- the length of time a person can be held under the section (duration),
- who can make the application or exercise the powers given under the section,
- the number of medical recommendations required, and
- the forms which must be completed.

	Maximum Duration	Application made by	No. of Medical Recommendations	Statutory Forms Required[a]
Section 2 Admission for Assessment	28 days		two	Forms 1 or 2 Forms 3 or 4 Forms 14 and 15
Section 4 Emergency Admission for Assessment	72 hours	Approved Social Worker or nearest relative	one	Forms 5 or 6 Forms 3 or 4 Forms 14 and 15
Section 3 Admission for Treatment	6 months[b]		two	Forms 8 or 9 Forms 10 or 11 Forms 14 and 15
		Power exercised by		
Section 5(2) Detention of In-patient	72 hours	Registered Medical Practitioner[c]	none	Forms 12 and 14
Section 5(4) Nurse's Holding Power	6 hours[d]	Prescribed Nurse	none	Forms 13 and 16

Notes

(a) Statutory MHA Forms for admission and records (see Appendix II for more detail).

(b) Can be renewed for a further six months and then for 12 months at a time.

(c) Registered medical practitioner in charge of patient's treatment or nominee.

(d) Or until earlier arrival of registered medical practitioner or nominee.

Reference should also be made to the Code of Practice issued by the Department of Health (see Chapter 2). The special case of patients referred from the courts or from prison is dealt with in Chapter 5 (Mentally disordered offenders).

Figure 4.1   **Overview of sections for compulsory detention under Part II of the Act.**

The exact wording of these sections is given in Appendix I(A). Reference should also be made to Appendix II of the Code of Practice issued by the Department of Health (see Chapter 2) and to Chapter 5 for the compulsory admission of patients referred from the courts or from prison.

**Section 2 –
admission for
assessment**

This is applicable where:

- the person is suffering from mental disorder of a nature or degree which warrants detention in a hospital for assessment (or for assessment followed by medical treatment) for at least a limited period, and
- he ought to be so detained in the interests of his health or safety or with a view to the protection of other persons.

Two medical recommendations are required under this section.

**Section 4 –
emergency
admission for
assessment**

The provisions here are as for section 2, but where seeking two medical recommendations would involve undesirable delay. Therefore only one is required, but preferably by a doctor who knows the patient.

**Section 3 –
admission for
treatment**

This is applicable where the behaviour of the patient warrants detention for treatment. Conditions for application for admission under section 3 are:

- that the mental disorder must be as defined by section 1(2) of the Act (see Chapter 3);
- that in cases of psychopathic disorder or mental impairment, treatment is likely to alleviate or prevent deterioration; and
- that treatment is necessary for the health or safety of the patient or for the protection of others and cannot be provided unless he is detained under this section.

The wording of section 3 is given in Appendix I(A).

**Section 5(2) –
detention of
informal patients**

This can be used in respect of in-patients to enable an application to be made for admission under section 2 or section 3. The registered medical practitioner furnishes to the hospital managers (see Chapter 19) a report that an application ought to be made for the admission of the patient under the Act. The patient may be detained in hospital for up to 72 hours from the time when the report is so furnished. Within that time a second doctor is called to examine the patient and an approved social worker to consider whether an application under section 2 or 3 should be made.

**Section 5(4) –
Nurse's Holding
Power**

This can be used in respect of in-patients receiving treatment for mental disorder where detention is necessary for the health or safety of the patient or protection of others and where it is not practicable to secure the attendance of the RMO. The wording of section 5(4) and 5(5) (dealing with records to be made) is given in Appendix I(A). For more detail on the Nurse's Holding Power see Part (4) below.

(3) Major implications for the nurse

Points of particular importance to the nurse are discussed below. The special case of the Nurse's Holding Power is discussed in Part (4).

Duration of the sections

It must be stressed that all the time limits set under the Act (see Figure 4.1) are maximum times within which appropriate steps must be taken to consider detention under another section or (in the case of section 3) to renew the section. If the patient ceases at any time to meet the requirements of the section of the Act under which he is detained, the RMO or hospital managers (see Chapter 19) have a duty to ensure that the section is terminated before the statutory time limit. Under section 2 (Admission for assessment), a patient can be detained **up to** 28 days. There is no provision to **renew** Section 2. If, following the assessment, it is considered that the patient requires admission as an in-patient for treatment, an application for admission under section 3 must be made before the expiry of section 2 (i.e. within the 28 days).

If a patient is detained under section 5(2) and, after an examination by another doctor and an approved social worker within the first 24 hours, it is decided that an application under the Act is not appropriate, the Section should end then (i.e. after the 24 hours). The patient then becomes 'informal' again and is not detained for the full 72 hours available under section 5(2).

Treatment

The general principle is that where possible the consent of the patient should be obtained before treatment is given. If however the patient is unable to give consent, or refuses to do so, and is detained compulsorily, treatment is possible under Part IV of the Act in defined circumstances (see Chapter 8, Consent to treatment).

Under section 2 – admission for assessment

Medication for mental disorder can be given compulsorily under section 63. ECT can be given only under section 58, unless the urgent provisions of section 62 apply.

Under section 4 – emergency admission for assessment

There is no provision in the Act for treatment to be given compulsorily. There is the possibility that treatment could be given under the powers at common law (see Chapter 8).

Under section 3 – admission for treatment

Where possible the patient's consent should be obtained before treatment is given. However compulsory medication for mental disorder can be given for the first three months under section 63. If the patient is incapable of giving consent or refuses to give consent a second opinion doctor (SOAD) must be brought in three months after medication was first given (section 58) unless the urgent provisions under section 62 apply. ECT can only be given with the consent of the patient or after a SOAD has been brought in (section 58) unless the urgent provisions under section 62 apply.

Informing the patient and nearest relative

Under section 2 (Admission for assessment) and section 3 (Admission for treatment)

The Mental Health Act 1983 leaflet for the appropriate section should be given to the patient and the information required under section 132 should also be explained to him by word of mouth (see Chapter 6). Because of changes in the patient's ability to understand this information, it is helpful to keep a record of the times at which the information is given and the level of understanding of the patient; and also for regular attempts to be made where it is clear that the patient has not understood it. A possible form (not a statutory form) is included in Appendix II, Example B. The managers (see Chapter 19) of the hospital or mental nursing home also have a **duty to advise the nearest relative** of the information given to the patient. This duty is set out in Chapter 6. The patient has the right to request that this information is **not** given to the nearest relative. In such cases it is useful to obtain this request in writing from the patient, but there is no statutory obligation to do so. Clearly, however, in the event of a subsequent dispute it is of advantage to have the patient's refusal in writing. Some hospitals provide a letter for the patient advising him of his right to refuse to allow the nearest relative to be notified.

Under section 4 (Admission for assessment in cases of emergency)

Even though the patient is only detained under this section for up to 72 hours there is still a duty upon the hospital managers to inform the patient of his rights. MHA 1983 Leaflet 2 should be given and the patient should also be told by word of mouth. If a second medical recommendation is obtained and section 2 commences it is then necessary to give the patient Leaflet 6 which applies to that section, even though it may only be a few hours since the information relevant to section 4 was given. The nearest relative also has to be informed of the patient's rights unless the patient has requested otherwise.

(4) Nurse's Holding Power

Section 5(4) of the Act gives to specific (prescribed) nurses the power to detain a patient who is an in-patient being treated for mental disorder in hospital if certain conditions are present. The detention can last for up to six hours or until the arrival of the RMO or his nominee within the six hours (see Appendix I(A), section 5(4)). Reference should also be made to Chapter 9 of the Code of Practice.

Who is the prescribed nurse?

The Mental Health (Nurses) Order 1983 (SI 1983 No. 891) (as amended by SI 1993 No. 2155) defines who are prescribed nurses for the purpose of section 5(4):

> a registered nurse in
> Part 3 (first level nurses trained in the nursing of persons suffering from mental illness) or
> Part 5 (first level nurses who are trained in the nursing of persons suffering from mental handicap) or
> Part 13 (nurses qualified following a course of preparation in mental health nursing) or
> Part 14 (nurses qualified following a course of preparation in mental handicap nursing)
> of the register prepared under section 10 of the Nurses, Midwives and Health Visitors Act 1979.

Reporting

The nurse has a duty under section 5(5) to deliver a record to the managers of the hospital as soon as possible after it is made. This duty should be carried out by her personally or by a person authorized by her.

Duration

If the nurse has made use of section 5(4) and the registered medical practitioner decides to use section 5(2), then the 72 hour period under that section begins with the time the nurse made out a report for the purposes of section 5(4) (see section 5(5)). Neither section 5(2) nor section 5(4) can be used in respect of an in-patient who is already liable to be detained under the Act (section 5(6)).

Informing the patient and nearest relative

Even though the Nurse's Holding Power lasts for a maximum of six hours and usually much less, there is still a statutory duty to inform the patient of his rights both in writing and by word of mouth. All that has been said in relation to informing the patient and the relatives for the other sections applies to section 5(4). Appendix II, Example A shows the relevant MHA 1983 Leaflet 1. Reference should also be made to Chapter 6.

Problems which have been encountered with section 5(4)

Q1. *Can any doctor attend on the informal patient as a result of the nurse using section 5(4)?*

A1. The doctor who is called must be the registered medical practitioner who is authorized to use section 5(2) or his nominee under section 5(3). That means he must be in charge of the treatment of the patient.

Q2. *If the doctor has not arrived before the six hours has expired could the nurse make another report under section 5(4) to prevent the patient leaving?*

A2. Whilst there is nothing in the Act which prohibits this it is entirely contrary to the spirit of the Act and the time limit of six hours. If the registered medical practitioner in charge of the treatment of the patient was unable to come for such a long time it might be possible for him to appoint a nominee under section 5(3) (see the Code of Practice, paragraph 9.8). Procedures should be devised which would prevent this possibility arising and ensure that the six hour period was adequate. The time limit for the comparable power of the nurse in Scotland is only two hours, and many would question why, given the rural nature of much of Scotland, six hours is necessary in England and Wales.

Q3. *How can the nurse restrain the patient?*

A3. Any reasonable methods would be possible, but clearly the least restrictive is essential. Reference should be made to Chapter 9 of the Code of Practice, paragraph 9.6).

Q4. *Can the patient be given compulsory medication?*

A4. Those patients detained under section 5(4) and 5(2) are outside the provisions of Part IV of the Act (Consent to Treatment) and therefore treatment cannot be given under the statutory provisions. In exceptional circumstances it might be possible to justify using common law powers, but the scope for such intervention against an unwilling person has not yet been judicially clarified (see Chapter 8).

Q5. *How long should the section be used?*

A5. The six hours is a maximum limit and in practice a much shorter time should be used. Research carried out by the author in Wales two years after the Act was implemented showed that in general only short periods were used, though there was one case where the doctor arrived only ten minutes before the six hours was due to expire.

Q6. *How could the use of the section be monitored?*

A6. It is possible to check on the use of section 5(4) by seeing how long it takes before the doctor arrives and the outcome in each case. Is a section 5(2) always used? If not, why not? Is section 5(4) being used appropriately?

Q7. *Would the use of section 5(4) interfere with the relationship of nurse to patient?*

A7. This was one of the fears which existed when the power was introduced. The fact that the nurse now had this statutory right was seen to affect the trust which should exist between nurse and patient. In practice this does not appear to have been the case, though clearly it depends upon how the nurse introduces it.

Q8. *What is the situation if the patient is in a general hospital and becomes mentally disordered?*

A8. Section 5(4) cannot be used unless the patient is an in-patient being treated for mental disorder. Thus, even though one of the nurses caring for the patient happened to be of the prescribed class, if the patient was being treated for a physical disorder section 5(4) would not apply. If a patient being treated for a physical condition becomes mentally disordered within the meaning of the Act (see Chapter 3) and it is considered essential that he should be prevented from leaving hospital it is possible for section 5(2) to be used by his doctor and a report made to the managers of the hospital. It is strongly recommended that, where the doctor is not a psychiatrist or a section 12 approved doctor, advice from such a doctor should be obtained. It would not be possible to transfer the patient to another hospital under different management on a section 5(2). Reference should be made to Chapter 8 of the Code of Practice, and to Practice Note Number 3 from the Mental Health Act Commission.

Arrangements must be made for the receipt by the managers of the medical report for the detention of the patient under section 5(2) and for the appropriate action then to be taken. Alternatively an application under section 4 could be made if there were an emergency situation and the requirements apart from two medical recommendations were satisfied. This would be the appropriate section if a patient admitted in an emergency to an accident and emergency department following a suicide attempt was considered to be mentally disordered within the meaning of the Act and satisfied the other requirements of section 4. Of course it is preferable to obtain a second medical recommendation and to admit the patient under section 2 or section 3.

Q9. *What about the situation in community homes for the mentally ill or mentally impaired?*

A9. For an in-patient to be detained under section 5(4) the home should be registered to take detained patients. In an emergency it might be necessary to use common law powers to prevent a patient leaving and being a danger to himself or to other people. In addition section 5(4) can only be used if a nurse of the prescribed class is on duty. Unfortunately not all community homes which are registered to take detained patients always have a nurse of the prescribed class on duty and this should be of concern to the registration authority.

(5) Renewal of section 3 – Admission for treatment

Within the period of two months ending on the day on which the patient would cease to be liable to detention, the RMO has a duty to examine the patient. If it appears to him that the required conditions (set out in section 20(4) – see Figure 4.2) are satisfied, he must furnish the managers of the hospital where the patient is detained with a report to that effect in the prescribed form (section 20(3)). This has the effect of detaining the patient for a further six months (initially) or 12 months (after the first renewal). The wording of section 20(3) is included in Appendix I(A).

(a) The patient is suffering from mental illness, severe mental impairment, psychopathic disorder or mental impairment, and his mental disorder is of a nature or degree which makes it appropriate for him to receive medical treatment in a hospital; and

(b) Such treatment is likely to alleviate or prevent a deterioration of his condition; and

(c) It is necessary for the health or safety of the patient or for the protection of other persons that he should receive such treatment and that it cannot be provided unless he continues to be detained.

Alternative condition (b) for those with mental illness or severe mental impairment:

(b) that the patient, if discharged, is unlikely to be able to care for himself, to obtain the care which he needs or to guard himself against serious exploitation.

Figure 4.2   Required conditions for renewal of section 3 – section 20(4).

Procedure to be followed in preparing a report for renewal

The RMO must consult one or more other persons who have been professionally concerned with the patient's medical treatment (section 20(5)). One of these persons will probably be the nurse caring for the patient. The nurse consulted should ensure that she keeps a record of her comments to the doctor. She must ensure that she understands the statutory basis for the renewal of the section (see Figure 4.2) and satisfy herself that she has a good knowledge of the patient's condition. The RMO does not have to accept her views. The importance of her record-keeping in this context cannot be over-emphasized.

Questions and exercises

(1) Obtain copies of all the forms used in the admission of a patient under (a) section 2, (b) section 3 and (c) section 4, and draw up a list of the differences.
NB. A listing of the forms can be found in Appendix II.

(2) Obtain sight of the statistics of patients under section 5(4) and section 5(2). What was the outcome for most patients?

(3) Analyse the statistics for compulsory admissions over the last year, what patterns can you see?

(4) A patient's records show that he was admitted under section 2 in

January then became informal. He was placed under section 2 again in May and then became informal and was placed on section 2 again in September. What questions would you ask about the appropriateness of the use of section 2 in these circumstances? Refer to Chapter 2 of the Code of Practice for further information on this.

Chapter 5   Admission to hospital under Part III of the Act: mentally disordered offenders

Part III of the Mental Health Act has the heading 'Patients concerned in Criminal Proceedings or under Sentence'. The provisions of Part III and the orders which can be made in relation to the mentally disordered offender form a difficult area for the nurse, especially as she may come across some of the sections only on rare occasions. However the nurse should ensure that she keeps up-to-date and is confident, since only then can she be sure that she can assist the patient with an understanding of his rights. She should also refer to Chapter 10 on leave of absence (section 17) since patients are sometimes transferred from an institution of high security to one of lower security under section 17 as part of a trial under the treatment plan. Details of the statutory provisions are set out in Figures 5.1 to 5.9.

Chapter 8 on consent to treatment is also very important since it deals with consent to treatment under Part IV of the Mental Health Act. Figure 5.10 towards the end of this chapter sets out which of the patients who have been involved in criminal proceedings and have been detained under Part III of the Act can be compulsorily treated under the provisions of Part IV of the Act.

Secure units

Special hospitals   There are three hospitals, Broadmoor, Rampton and Ashworth (formerly Park Lane and Moss-side), which provide conditions of high security. They come under the control of the Special Hospitals Health Authority. They are funded at present directly from the Home Office. In the early 1990s an inquiry into Ashworth chaired by Sir Louis Blom-Cooper following complaints by relatives and patients recommended major reforms. The Government subsequently set up a panel of specialists to make recommendations on the future of the special hospitals.

At present the system of funding is a direct disincentive to purchasers to arrange for the transfer of patients from the special hospitals if they need continued secure accommodation, since the patients are likely to require accommodation costing the purchaser between £70 000 to £100 000 per year. From April 1996 each special hospital will be managed by a special health authority with new purchasing arrangements.

Regional secure units

In most regions there exists a regional unit providing greater security than that usually provided within a psychiatric hospital. Some of these are funded through top-slicing (see Glossary) of the region's allocation for health services. Increasingly however the costs of the places are falling on individual NHS purchasers.

Reed Reports

In 1991 a review of the health and social services for mentally disordered offenders and others requiring similar services was conducted under the chairmanship of Dr John Reed. Consultation documents on the recommendations of its three advisory groups: prison advisory group, hospital advisory group, and community advisory group and the overview of the steering committee were circulated for discussion.

Additional working parties on high security and related psychiatric provision and also on psychopathic disorder were also set up, both chaired by Dr John Reed, and reported in 1994. Action upon their recommendations is currently awaited.

Funding for special projects for the mentally disordered offender now exist in many areas and some have a sophisticated diversion scheme in operation to prevent the person being sent to prison when alternative care and treatment is required.

Legal options for mentally disordered offenders (summary)

The mental capacity or condition of an accused person or offender can become an issue at many different stages. The various legal possibilities are given in summary below.

Initially it may be that an individual is thought unfit to plead or be tried before the court. If this is so, special arrangements exist as a result of the Criminal Procedure (Insanity) Act 1964 and its recent amendments in the 1991 Act. These are discussed below. These acts also cover the circumstances where the accused may be held fit to plead but he defends himself on the basis that at the time that the alleged offence was committed he was insane.

In some cases, the court may decide, sometimes before sentencing and in other cases after sentencing, that the accused should be sent to a psychiatric hospital in order that he can be assessed or given treatment. The various orders which are then available and the stages at which these can be made, by whom and on what basis are discussed below.

Even when the patient is transferred to custodial care, on remand or after sentencing the Home Secretary has the power to transfer him to a psychiatric hospital.

Procedure under the Criminal Procedure (Insanity) Act 1964 as amended by the Criminal Procedure (Insanity and Unfitness to Plead) Act 1991

Not guilty by reason of insanity

The 1964 Act enables an acquittal to be recorded on grounds of insanity. The wording is: 'The accused is not guilty by reason of insanity'. Insanity is defined by the courts according to the M'Naghten rules laid down in the 19th century (see Glossary) and relates to the state of mind of the accused at the time of the offence.

Unfit to plead

The 1964 Act also enables the court to find that the accused is not capable of understanding the trial process and an order can be made that the accused be admitted to such hospital as may be specified by the Secretary of State subject to restriction without limit of time.

The 1991 Act amendments

There were considerable limitations to the 1964 Act in relation to the possibility that the accused was not guilty of the offence he was accused of, the outcomes available to the court, and the medical evidence on which the court based its decision.

The 1991 Act which came into force on 1 January 1992 introduced the following changes.

A trial of facts

It is now possible for there to be a trial of facts where an accused is found unfit to be tried. In this way the jury can decide if it is satisfied beyond reasonable doubt that the accused did the act or made the omission charged against him. This prevents a situation arising where a person is subject to an order under the Act on the grounds that he is not fit to stand trial, when a defence could have been produced to show that he did not commit the offence with which he is charged. Even if the accused is transferred to hospital without trial, if it subsequently becomes possible to have a trial of the facts there can be a court hearing for this to take place.

Disposals

The range of disposals open to the courts now include:

- detention in hospital with or without a restriction order,
- guardianship order,
- supervision in the community, and
- absolute discharge.

Medical evidence

The jury cannot return a verdict of not guilty by reason of insanity nor can the accused be found unfit to plead, unless evidence is given by two or more medical practitioners, at least one of whom is duly approved under section 12 of the Act .

What are the effects on patients sent to hospital under the 1964 Act (as amended)?

The patient is treated as though he were sent under section 37 with or without restrictions. He is however entitled to apply to a Mental Health Review Tribunal in the first six months of detention instead of having to wait for the second six months (section 69(2)).

Court orders in relation to mental disorder

There is a wide range of options open to the court if it appears that the accused is suffering from mental disorder. The 1983 Act increased the range of options available by enabling the court to order the detention of the accused, before trial or after conviction, in a hospital for psychiatric care.

The powers of the court vary according to:

- the legal situation of the patient (before or after trial);
- the type of court (i.e. magistrates' or crown court);
- the nature of the medical evidence; and
- the nature of the offence with which the defendant is charged or convicted.

What follows is a brief summary of the orders which are available, the conditions which must exist before the orders can be made and the effect of the orders. Appendix I(A) gives headings and extracts from the relevant sections. Figure 5.1 sets out the orders available.

Section 35	–	remand for reports
Section 36	–	remand for treatment
Section 37	–	hospital order (with or without a restriction order under section 41 (see below)
Section 38	–	interim hospital order

Figure 5.1 Orders available to the criminal courts.

Figures 5.2 to 5.5 give more detail of duration, court/offence, medical criteria, and administrative criteria applicable to orders under sections 35, 36, 37 and 38.

Section 35 – remand for report
28 days, renewable for up to another 28 days up to a maximum of 12 weeks in all. (The further remands can be made by the courts without the presence of accused in court provided he is legally represented in court.)

Section 36 – remand for treatment
28 days at a time. Maximum of 12 weeks in all. (Further remands by court as for section 35.)

Section 37 – hospital or guardianship order*
Six months, renewable for another six months and then for a year at a time.

Section 38 – interim hospital order
Up to six weeks renewable for 28 days at a time up to a maximum of six months in all. If an interim order is made the court can make the hospital order without the accused appearing in court provided that he is legally represented.

Section 47 – transfer direction (those under sentence)*
The duration is as for a hospital order section 37. This means that a person could be kept in hospital beyond the date at which he would have been released, had he remained in prison.

A transfer direction ceases to have effect at the expiration of 14 days beginning with the day on which it is given unless within that period the person with respect to whom it was given has been received into the hospital specified in the direction.

Section 48 – transfer direction (other prisoners)*
Similar provisions to section 47.

*Note A restriction order (section 41) can be placed by the courts on a hospital order section 37, and a restriction direction (section 49) can be placed by the Secretary of State on a transfer under section 47 or section 48. These are explained below.

Figure 5.2 Orders made by the court and transfers from prison – duration.

Section 35 – remand for report
Crown court awaiting trial for offence punishable with imprisonment or has been arraigned but not yet dealt with. Cannot use order if convicted of offence punishable by sentence fixed by law (i.e. murder).

Magistrates' court
(a) if convicted of offence punishable with imprisonment, or
(b) if charged with such an offence and court is satisfied that he did the act or made the omission, or
(c) if Defendant has consented to section 35 order.

Section 36 – remand for treatment
Awaiting trial before crown court for an offence punishable with imprisonment (where sentence not fixed by law) or who is in custody in course of trial.

Section 37 – hospital or guardianship order
Magistrates' and Crown Court after conviction. Magistrates' Court pre-conviction if court is satisfied that the accused did the act or made the omission charged. Offence punishable with imprisonment (where sentence is not fixed by law).

Section 38 – interim hospital order
Person convicted before the Crown or Magistrates' Court of offence punishable with imprisonment (except where fixed by law).

Figure 5.3 Orders made by the court – Court/Offence.

Section 35 – remand for report
Written or oral evidence of one registered medical practitioner that there is reason to suspect accused person is suffering from mental illness, psychopathic disorder, severe mental impairment or mental impairment.

Further remands must be based on written or oral evidence that it is necessary for completing the assessment of accused's mental condition.

Section 36 – remand for treatment
Written or oral evidence of two registered medical practitioners that defendant is suffering from mental illness or severe mental impairment of a nature which makes it appropriate for him to be detained in a hospital for medical treatment.

Further remands if it appears to court on written or oral evidence of the RMO that it is warranted.

Section 37 – hospital or guardianship order
Written or oral evidence of two registered medical practitioners that offender is suffering from mental illness, psychopathic disorder, severe mental impairment or mental impairment and either

- the mental disorder is of a nature or degree which makes it appropriate for him to be detained in hospital for medical treatment and in case of psychopathic disorder or mental impairment such treatment is likely to alleviate or prevent a deterioration of his condition, or
- the offender is over 16 years of age and his mental disorder is of a nature or degree which warrants his reception into guardianship under the Act.

Section 38 – interim hospital order
Written or oral evidence of two registered medical practitioners (one of whom must be section 12 approved) that

- the offender is suffering from mental illness, psychopathic disorder, severe mental impairment, or mental impairment; and
- there is reason to suppose that the mental disorder is such that it may be appropriate for a hospital order to be made.

Section 47 – transfer direction (those under sentence)
Reports by at least two registered medical practitioners

- that the person is suffering from mental illness, psychopathic disorder, severe mental impairment or mental impairment; and
- that the mental disorder from which that person is suffering is of a nature or degree which makes it appropriate for him to be detained in a hospital for medical treatment; and
- (in the case of psychopathic disorder or mental impairment) that such treatment is likely to alleviate or prevent a deterioration of his condition.

Section 48 – transfer direction (other prisoners e.g. on remand, committed by civil court, Immigration Act detainees)
The Secretary of State must be satisfied by the same reports as are required for the purposes of section 47 above that

- that person is suffering from mental illness or severe mental impairment of a nature or degree which makes it appropriate for him to be detained in a hospital for medical treatment, **and**
- that he is in urgent need of such treatment.

The Secretary of State shall have the same power of giving a transfer direction in respect of him as if he were serving a sentence of imprisonment.

Figure 5.4 Orders made by the court and transfers from prison – medical criteria.

Section 35 – remand for report

Written or oral evidence of registered medical practitioner who would be responsible for making a report or of representative of managers of hospital that arrangements have been made for admission to hospital within seven days from date of remand.

Section 36 – remand for treatment

Written or oral evidence of satisfactory arrangements for admission to hospital within seven days of remand – as for section 35 above.

Section 37 – hospital or guardianship order

Court satisfied on written or oral evidence of

- the registered medical practitioner who would be in charge of the treatment or
- some other person representing the manager of the hospital

that arrangements have been made for his admission to that hospital in the event of such an order being made by the court and for his admission to it within the period of 28 days beginning with the date of the making of such an order. Pending admission within 28 days, the court can give direction for conveyance to and detention in a place of safety.

Section 38 – interim hospital order

Written or oral evidence of satisfactory arrangements for admission to hospital within 28 days of date of order – as for section 37.

Section 47 – transfer direction (those under sentence)

A transfer direction ceases to have effect at the expiration of 14 days beginning with the day on which it is given unless within that period the person with respect to whom it was given has been received into the hospital specified in the direction.

The direction must specify the form of mental disorder from which the person is suffering and the medical recommendations must refer to the same disorder, whether or not they refer to additional ones. The transfer cannot be made to a mental nursing home. The practice has developed of transferring a person to an NHS hospital and then to a private nursing home with secure facilities.

Section 48 – transfer direction (other prisoners)

As for section 47.

Figure 5.5 Orders made by the court and transfers from prison – administrative criteria.

Restriction order

Where the crown court directs that the defendant should be subject to a hospital order, this can be linked with a restriction order under section 41. The effect of this restriction order is that the patient comes under the control of the Home Secretary. The hospital managers and the responsible medical officer (RMO) do not have the powers which they have over a patient subject simply to detention under section 37. The main provisions are set out below in Figure 5.6.

Restrictions
These include:

- exclusion of provisions relating to duration, renewal and expiration of authority to detain;
- no application to MHRT in first six months; and
- Secretary of State retains powers over leave of absence, transfer and discharge under section 23.

Duration
Unlimited or period specified by the Crown Court after conviction.

Offences
As for section 37.

Medical criteria
As for hospital order (section 37) but one of the two registered medical practitioners must give evidence orally to court.

Judicial criteria
That it is necessary for the protection of the public from serious harm having regard to:

- the nature of the offence
- the antecedents of the offender, and
- the risk of his committing further offences if set at large.

The court may further order that offender be subject to special restrictions.

Figure 5.6   Restriction orders – section 41.

Transfers from prison

Even where the defendant has been transferred to prison, whether on remand before trial or sentencing, or after conviction and sentencing, the Home Secretary can transfer the person to a hospital for treatment. Details are shown in Figures 5.7 to 5.9. Section 47 enables the Secretary of State to arrange for of a

Figure 5.7 Removal to hospital of persons serving sentences of imprisonment – section 47.

Who is covered?

- Persons detained as a result of court sentence or order for detention by court in criminal proceedings.
- Persons committed to custody under section 115(3) of Magistrates Act (failure to keep the peace etc.).
- Persons committed to prison for failure to pay fine.

Figure 5.8 Transfer of prisoners other than those covered by section 47 – section 48.

Who is covered?

- Persons detained in a prison or remand centre, not being persons serving a sentence of imprisonment or those covered below.
- Persons remanded in custody by a magistrates' court.
- Civil prisoners.
- Persons detained under the Immigration Act 1971.

Figure 5.9 Restriction direction – section 49.

The Secretary of State may, if he thinks fit, direct that the person under a transfer direction shall be subject to special restrictions set out in section 41.

The responsible medical officer must examine the person under a restriction direction and make reports to the Secretary of State as often as he directs and not less that once per year.

person serving a sentence of imprisonment to be transferred to a hospital and section 48 enables the transfer of other prisoners to be made.

Judgement is exercised by the Secretary of State. If he is satisfied of the medical criteria (see Figure 5.4), he may by warrant direct that the person be removed to and detained at such hospital (not being a mental nursing home) as may be specified in the direction. The direction is known as a transfer direction.

Duration, medical criteria, and administrative criteria are given in Figures 5.2, 5.4 and 5.5.

Restriction direction

Where the Home Secretary orders the transfer of a person from prison to a psychiatric hospital, the transfer can be made subject to a restriction direction under section 49. Thus section 47 and section 48 are usually linked with restrictions under section 49.

Section 49 operates in a similar manner to section 41 and details are given in Figure 5.9.

Further provisions – section 50

If a direction under section 47 has been made (with a restriction under section 49) and, before the person's prison sentence would have expired, the Secretary of State is informed that the person no longer requires treatment in hospital, the Secretary of State may:

- direct his transfer to any prison or institution in which he could have been detained had he not been transferred to hospital; or
- exercise any power of releasing him on licence or discharging him under supervision which would have been exercisable if he had been remitted to such prison or institution.

Following the arrival of the person in prison or other institution, the transfer direction and the restriction direction shall cease to have effect.

Once the time of a person's sentence would have expired, the restriction direction shall cease to have effect (section 50(2)).

Further provisions are dealt with in section 51 (detained persons), section 52 (those remanded by magistrates' courts), section 53 (civil prisoners and those detained under the Immigration Act 1971) and section 54 (requirements as to medical evidence).

Treatment of mentally disordered offenders

Figure 5.10 sets out which patients who have been involved in criminal proceedings and have been detained under Part III of

Part IV treatment provisions cover the following Part III patients:

Section 36 – Those remanded for treatment.
Section 37 – Those under a hospital order or guardianship with or without a restriction order under section 41.
Section 38 – Those under interim hospital orders.
Section 47 – Those serving sentence and removed to hospital.
Section 48 – Other prisoners removed to hospital.

Also those patients transferred under the provisions of the Criminal Procedure (Insanity) Act 1964 (as amended). Details of the amendments are given earlier in this chapter.

Figure 5.10 Offenders covered by Part IV treatment provisions.

the Act can be compulsorily treated under the provisions of Part IV of the Act.

Important points to note

As we can see from Figures 5.1 to 5.10, the situation regarding mentally disordered offenders is complex. Important points for the nurse are:

(1) If in doubt always check in the notes the sections under which a patient is held.

(2) Once the section is known criteria relevant for this patient can be checked in Figures 5.2 to 5.5 and/or in the Act itself.

(3) Patients under section 35 (remand for reports) may **not** be given treatment compulsorily under Part IV of the Act.

(4) Section 37 (the hospital order) is comparable to section 3 (admission for treatment) except there is no right of the nearest relative to discharge and no application to a Mental Health Review Tribunal within the first six months. The patient and the nearest relative do have the right to apply to an MHRT in the second six months.

(5) Patients under restriction orders and directions are under the jurisdiction of the Secretary of State.

Questions and exercises

(1) What provisions exist to deal with the mentally disordered offender?

(2) A patient is transferred to psychiatric hospital from prison under section 47, what rights does he have? What differences would there be if the patient was also subject to a restriction direction under section 49?

(3) A patient is sent to hospital by the court under section 35. Could he be compelled to have treatment under Part IV of the Act?

(4) An informal patient attacks another patient causing severe injuries, what is the policy on the notification of such an incident to the police?

Chapter 6 Provision of information to the patient and nearest relative

A great deal of information must be provided to the detained patient and to the nearest relative. The information that must be provided is summarized in Figure 6.1. Reference should also be made to Chapter 14 of the Code of Practice.

On admission

- Reasons for detention
- Implications of sections under which detained
- Rights to apply to the Mental Health Review Tribunal (MHRT)
- Rights of nearest relative to discharge
- Consent to treatment provisions
- Procedures for complaints
- Rules for correspondence
- Right to appeal to the managers

Other

- Information about treatment
- Right of access to records
- Information to nearest relative of intended discharge

Figure 6.1 Summary of information to be provided to the patient and nearest relative.

This chapter gives greater detail on **what** information is to be provided and discusses **when**, **how** and **by whom** it should be given and the records that should be kept.

Information to detained patients

The managers have a statutory responsibility to give information to the detained patient under section 132.

***What* information must be given?**

This is summarized in Figure 6.2.

(1) The provisions of the Mental Health Act 1983 under which the patient is detained and the effect of those provisions.

(2) What rights of applying to an MHRT exist for him for the section he is under.

(3) The effect of sections 23 and 25 (i.e. the right of the nearest relative to discharge the patient on giving 72 hours notice, subject to a report advising against discharge by the Responsible Medical Officer (RMO)); the rights of discharge of the RMO and the managers.

(4) The effect of the consent to treatment provisions.

(5) The right to apply to an MHRT where an order for discharge has been made unsuccessfully by the nearest relative under section 23.

(6) The duty of the Secretary of State to prepare a Code of Practice.

(7) The duty of the Secretary of State to keep under review the exercise of powers under the Act and to arrange for detained patients to be visited and their complaints investigated, and that these functions have been delegated to the Mental Health Act Commission (MHAC).

(8) The rules relating to correspondence.

Figure 6.2 Information which must be given to the detained patient.

When should the information be given?

The Act requires that steps should be taken as soon as practicable to ensure that the patient understands the above provisions and as soon as possible after the patient is detained under the Act. Since the patient may well be too distressed to understand the information initially, it is important that the information is repeated until the patient understands, since that is the statutory requirement. No form has officially been prepared for recording the giving of information to the patient and the level of the patient's understanding, but a suggested one is shown in Appendix II, Example B.

Every time the patient is placed under a section, the information must be given, both in writing and by word of mouth.

How must the information be given?

The steps must include the giving of information both by word of mouth and in writing. There are government leaflets relating to the different sections (see Appendix II, Example A for the leaflet relevant to section 5(4)) and some translations are now available. Since the aim is to ensure that the patient **under-**

stands, any disability must be taken int⸍ arrangements must be made for those who ⸍ who do not understand English. Interpreters⸍ even if translated leaflets are available sin⸍ must be given by word of mouth as well.

Who should give the information?

The duty is on the managers to make arrangements for the giving of this information. It is a duty which can be delegated and therefore a procedure should be drawn up which sets out:

- who should have the responsibility of giving the information,
- how the giving of information should be recorded,
- how to include in the records the level of the patient's understanding,
- arrangements for repeating the giving of information, and
- arrangements for monitoring that the procedure is being implemented.

Ultimately the managers have the legal responsibility of ensuring that the requirements of the Act are met.

What is the nurse's involvement?

The nurse is likely to be one of the professionals to whom the task of informing the patient is delegated. It may be that the procedure gives the responsibility to the nurses on the ward. It is preferable for there to be an individual decision in relation to each patient since certain staff may find it easier to ensure that the patient understands. Sometimes the procedure gives the task to the Patient Services Officer. However it is important that there should be provision for evenings and weekends when administrative staff are not on duty, since there is no justification in delaying the giving of information until administrative staff are available.

If the nurse is aware that she does not have a good relationship with a particular patient, then she might suggest that another more appropriate person takes over the task.

The nurse is often the most in touch with the detained patient and, if she is aware from the patient's questions that the patient still does not understand some of the legal provisions, she should ensure that the relevant information is given again and recorded. Even when the information has been given and is understood, it is good practice to arrange for the information to be given again at regular intervals.

Complaints

Detained patients have the right to complain to the MHAC if the hospital managers have not answered satisfactorily. A direct complaint to the MHAC can be made by anyone in relation to the use of powers or carrying out duties under the Act (see Chapter 20).

Which patients are not covered by these provisions?

The above statutory provisions do not cover those patients who are under guardianship nor those who are detained under section 136 in a place other than a hospital such as a police station. However there is no reason why in practice they should not be given as much information as possible and procedures should be set up to that effect. The provisions of the Police and Criminal Evidence Act 1984 will apply to a patient taken by the police to a police station as a place of safety under section 136 (see Chapter 13).

Information to informal patients

Informal patients have no rights to be given information under the Act except in relation to brain surgery for mental disorder or hormonal implants for reducing sex drive (section 57).

However, even though there is no duty under the Mental Health legislation, good practice would mean ensuring that they are kept fully informed about the progress of plans for their care and treatment. In addition the Patient's Charter states that patients should be given information about the hospital and its facilities and many hospitals now have information booklets and their own charters.

Information about the complaints procedure

All patients should receive information relating to the complaints procedure and the name of the designated officer for complaints. This is a statutory requirement under the Hospital Complaints Procedure Act 1985.

Information about treatment

Where treatment is being discussed, patients are entitled to receive information relevant to their consent. The patient should receive such information as would be given by a doctor following the standards of the reasonable professional (the Bolam test). This is the common law position which is set out by the House of Lords in *Sidaway* v. *Board of Governors of Bethlem Royal Hospital* (1985) (see Glossary). The book *Patients' Rights, Responsibilities and the Nurse* (Dimond, 1993) is a good source of further information.

Some hospitals have devised information leaflets which describe the medication and its side effects in language which can be clearly understood by non-medical people.

Access to health records

There is also a statutory right of access to health records under the Access to Health Records Act 1990 which came into force on 1 November 1991. This applies to all patients, detained and informal. There is a power of exclusion of the right of access where it would cause serious harm to the physical or mental health of the patient or a third person, or where the identity of a third person who did not wish to be identified would be made known. The important point is that any exclusion of access to information must be done on an individual patient basis and justified individually; it is not possible for there to be a blanket policy for example that no patients on 'Y' ward can have access to their records or no detained patient can have access.

The right of access applies not only to the daily medical and nursing records but also to those reports which are prepared by healthcare professionals for an MHRT or managers' hearing. If a health professional is of the view that serious harm would be caused to the physical or mental well-being of the patient should all or part of the report be disclosed, those parts which should be withheld should be clearly marked and the health professional must be prepared to justify the withholding.

The Mental Health Review Tribunal Rules 1983 (SI 1983 No. 942) also include the right to withhold information from the patient in appropriate circumstances. However this should be exceptional.

Information to the nearest relative

The nearest relative or the person appearing to the managers to be the nearest relative has a statutory right to be given the same written information that the patient receives on admission, unless the patient requests otherwise.

Information on detention of the patient

The managers must take such steps as are practical for this to be given to the nearest relative when the patient receives the information or within a reasonable period of time thereafter.

If the patient has been detained under section 2, the nearest relative should already have been informed by the approved social worker of the application or the intended application (section 11(3)). The approved social worker has to inform the nearest relative of the nearest relative's power under section 23(2)(a) to order a discharge. If the patient has been detained under section 3 or guardianship, then the nearest relative should have been consulted under section 11(4) before the application was made. Such consultation can be dispensed with if in the circumstances it is not reasonably practicable or would involve unreasonable delay. In most cases however the nearest relative would know of the patient's admission.

The managers do not have a statutory duty to ensure that the nearest relative **understands** the information supplied, nor does the information have to be given by word of mouth. However where it is known that the nearest relative is not English speaking or is suffering from a disability, every effort should be made to provide translation of the statutory information or facilities for those who are disabled.

Information about intended discharge

The managers have a duty under section 133 to take such steps as are practicable to inform the nearest relative of the patient's discharge. This information, if practicable, should be given at least seven days before the date of discharge. This requirement also applies to patients detained under section 4 and section 5(2) but in such cases there cannot be seven days' notice.

Information *not* to be given to the nearest relative

The patient can request that the nearest relative should **not** be given the written information on detention or of the proposed discharge. In addition, the nearest relative can request not to receive notification of the discharge. Both these provisions can cause difficulties. In particular if the after-care provisions for the patient depend upon the care of the nearest relative then keeping the nearest relative in ignorance can cause considerable problems. In many cases however, if discharge has been planned since admission under the section 117 provisions, it is likely that the nearest relative would have been involved at an earlier date.

Similarly if the nearest relative has reason to be fearful of the patient's discharge, the right of the patient to prevent this information being passed on can cause difficulties. However it is a statutory right of the patient to request that the information be withheld.

Where the patient has made a request that the information should not be passed on (whether when the detention begins or when discharge is planned) it is advisable to record this request in writing in case there is any subsequent dispute. Forms should be available. Some hospitals have designed their own forms where the patient signs that he does not wish the nearest relative to be informed (see Appendix II, Example B).

Questions and exercises

(1) A patient is admitted in an emergency for assessment (section 4), is then detained under section 2 and then detained for treatment under section 3. Outline the information which would have to be given by word of mouth and in writing on each occasion. How would you record this and what procedures would you follow to ensure the giving of information was repeated when necessary?

(2) What special steps would you take in giving the statutory information in the following circumstances:

- the patient is deaf,
- the patient is blind,
- the patient is severely mentally handicapped,
- the patient is 15 years old,
- the patient refuses to listen, or
- the patient is Indian.

(3) The patient has asked that the nearest relative is not informed about his detention. The nearest relative arrives on the ward and complains to you about not being informed of the detention. What action would you take?

(4) Look at a leaflet included in Appendix II for giving information to the patient (Example A). How clear do you think it is? What additional information do you consider you would have to give the patient by word of mouth in order that the patient has a full understanding of his rights?

Chapter 7   The nearest relative

Statutory definitions

Section 26

Considerable significance and powers are given by the Mental Health Act 1983 to the nearest relative. The definition was widened compared with the 1959 Mental Health Act to ensure that it is more meaningful in terms of those likely to be closest to the patient. The definition and the order of priority is shown in Figure 7.1.

---

(1) Any relative with whom the patient ordinarily resides or who cares for him (section 26(4))

(2) Husband or wife (includes a person living as the husband or wife for at least six months)(section 26(6))

(3) Son or daughter

(4) Father or mother

(5) Brother or sister

(6) Grandparent

(7) Grandchild

(8) Uncle or aunt

(9) Nephew or niece

A person **other than a relative**, with whom the patient ordinarily resides and has done so for a period of not less than five years (section 26(7)). (This person may go to the top of the order of priority unless a relative who comes higher in the hierarchy is also living with the patient.)

Notes

(a) Any relationship of the half-blood shall be treated as a relationship of the whole blood and an illegitimate person shall be treated as the legitimate child of his mother.

(b) In determining priority relatives of the whole blood are preferred to relatives of the half-blood.

(c) The elder or eldest of two or more relatives in the same category are preferred to the other(s) of those relatives regardless of sex.

Figure 7.1 Definition of the nearest relative in order of priority – section 26.

The Children Act 1989

Where the patient is a child or young person in the care of the local authority by virtue of a care order under the Children Act 1989, then that Act provides that the authority shall be deemed the nearest relative of the patient in preference to any person except the patient's husband or wife (Children Act 1989, Schedule 13, paragraph 48).

Where a guardian has been appointed for a person who has not attained the age of eighteen years, or a residence order is in force with respect to such a person, then the guardian (or guardians if there is more than one), shall, to the exclusion of any other person, be deemed to be his nearest relative.

Disregard of certain persons for the definition of nearest relative

Certain persons are disregarded for the purposes of the definition of nearest relative. These are listed in Figure 7.2.

Figure 7.2 Persons disregarded for the purposes of defining the nearest relative – section 26(5).

- A non-resident of the UK, Channel Islands or Isle of Man (where the patient is so resident).
- The husband or wife who is permanently separated or has deserted or been deserted by the patient.
- A person not being the husband, wife, father or mother who is under 18 years.
- A person subject to an order under section 38 of the Sexual Offences Act 1956 which divests him of authority over the patient.

Powers of the nearest relative

The powers and duties of the nearest relative are set out in Figure 7.3.

The nearest relative has to be informed of certain information though the patient can request that the information is not passed on. Details of this are given in Chapter 6.

Discharge by the nearest relative

This right applies to the nearest relatives of patients under sections 2 and 3 and also to guardianship. Where the patient is detained in hospital the nearest relative must give to the managers 72 hours' notice in writing of his intention to discharge the patient. It is assumed that the 72 hours would run from the time that the managers receive the notice in writing. In the case of guardianship, the notice would go to the local social services authority.

In the case of a patient liable to be detained in hospital, within

(1) Application for admission of the patient under:

- section 2 for assessment,
- section 3 for treatment, or
- section 4 – emergency admission for assessment.

(2) Application for the patient to be placed under guardianship section 7.

(3) Must be consulted by the approved social worker and can object to an application by an approved social worker for the patient's admission for treatment or for a guardianship order.

(4) Must be notified of any application for admission for assessment and in an emergency – sections 2 and 4.

(5) Can discharge the patient under section 23 after giving to the managers 72 hours' notice of such an intention (see below).

(6) Can authorize a registered medical practitioner at any reasonable time to visit and examine the patient in private. The doctor can also require the production of any records relating to the detention or treatment of the patient in any hospital and inspect them (section 24(1) and (2).

(7) Can apply to a Mental Health Review Tribunal (MHRT) on the occasions set out in Figure 9.4.

Figure 7.3 Powers and duties of a nearest relative.

the 72 hours the responsible medical officer (RMO) has the power to recommend that the nearest relative's order is overruled.

If the RMO furnishes to the managers a report certifying that in his opinion the patient, if discharged, would be likely to act in a manner dangerous to other persons or to himself, two consequences follow:

- the order for discharge made by the nearest relative shall have no effect, and
- no further order for the discharge of the patient shall be made by that relative during the period of six months beginning with the date of the report.

The managers must ensure that the nearest relative is notified of the report and its outcome (section 25(2)). The nearest relative has a right of appeal to the MHRT if the patient is detained under section 3 and the RMO has barred the discharge by the nearest relative.

There are no time limits set on the notification by the managers to the nearest relative under section 25(2) but one would assume that it should be as soon as is reasonably practicable.

Removal of the nearest relative and/or appointment of replacement

Since the nearest relative can have such an important part to play in the patient's protection, it is essential that where the nearest relative is not acting in the best interests of the patient or where there is no known nearest relative then either the nearest relative should be replaced or a new person appointed.

Grounds for taking action

Grounds for appointing an acting nearest relative are set out in Figure 7.4.

> (1) That the patient has no nearest relative within the meaning of the Act, or that it is not reasonably practicable to ascertain whether he has such a relative or who that relative is.
>
> (2) That the nearest relative of the patient is incapable of acting as such by reason of mental disorder or other illness.
>
> (3) That the nearest relative of the patient unreasonably objects to the making of an application for admission for treatment or a guardianship application in respect of the patient.
>
> (4) That the nearest relative of the patient has exercised without due regard to the welfare of the patient or the interests of the public his power to discharge the patient from hospital or guardianship or is likely to do so.

Figure 7.4
Appointment by court of acting nearest relative – section 29(3).

The grounds shown in Figure 7.4 do not cover all eventualities. There is some concern that in some cases the nearest relative may not be acting in the best interests of the patient but it is not possible under these provisions to replace that person unless he is objecting to the admission or seeking the discharge.

For example the nearest relative may be the father of a patient over 18 years and the patient may allege he has abused her but, unless that father comes within the provisions for disqualification set out in Figure 7.4, it would not be possible to obtain an order for a replacement. Reform of this to give a discretionary power to the court when it is in the best interests of the patient has been suggested (see *Fourth Biennial Report of the Mental Health Act Commission 1989–1990*).

Procedure for appointment of an acting nearest relative

If the grounds set out in Figure 7.4 apply a court application should be initiated. If the nurse is aware that a patient does not appear to have a nearest relative it may be appropriate for her to suggest to the approved social worker that an application should be made for one to be appointed. The nurse can tell from looking at the statutory documentation for admission, whether the approved social worker was able to consult with the nearest relative before the application was made or whether the nearest relative was not known or did not appear to exist. Since the nearest relative has such wide powers there are considerable advantages to the patient in ensuring that one is appointed. The procedure which is followed is shown in Figure 7.5.

The application for the appointment of an acting nearest relative is not considered to be finally disposed of until the time for an appeal has expired or the appeal been heard or withdrawn.

Application
An application must be made to the county court by one of the following:

- any relative of the patient;
- any other person with whom the patient is residing or was last residing with pre-admission; or
- an approved social worker

Who can be appointed?
The county court can order that the function of the nearest relative shall be exercisable by:

- the applicant;
- by any other person specified in the application being a person who, in the opinion of the court, is a proper person to act as the patient's nearest relative and is willing to do so; or
- in the case of an application by an approved social worker, the local social services authority

Extension of detention period – section 29(4)
If before the application to the county court the patient is liable to be detained under an admission for assessment (i.e. section 2), then the period of detention is extended:

- until the application under this section has been finally disposed of; and
- if an order is made under this section, for a further period of seven days.

Figure 7.5 Procedure for the appointment of an acting nearest relative – section 29.

There is a danger that a prolonged delay waiting for the application to come before the county court could mean that the patient remains under section 2 for much longer than would otherwise be permitted. If this occurs it is possible to seek an order from the High Court to speed up the hearing of the application. The County Court Rules and regulations issued by the Secretary of State prescribe the manner in which certain acts are to be performed and set the detailed procedures.

The nearest relative can authorize someone else to act as nearest relative but it must be in writing Regulation 14 of the Mental Health (Hospital, Guardianship and Consent to Treatment) Regulations 1983 (SI 1983 No. 893).

The nearest relative and the informal patient

The above discussion relates to the nearest relative of the detained patient. However even when the patient is informal there are considerable advantages to be obtained from ensuring that maximum contact is maintained with those relatives and friends closest to the patient. The statutory definitions do not have to be followed and if a relative or friend who would not constitute the nearest relative under the Act is the person most inclined to visit the patient and keep in contact with him, then this link should be encouraged and the relationship supported. However it must be remembered that, should this occur and then the patient has to be detained, this person will not necessarily be the nearest relative for the purposes of the Act.

Under section 117, patients detained under certain sections **must** have planned after-care (see Chapter 17). All other patients, whether detained or informal, benefit considerably from the involvement of their friends and relatives in the treatment plan and care plans for after discharge. There is much benefit to be derived in staff and managers encouraging the establishment of local support groups and in having leaflets available for distribution to relatives and friends about local and national self-help carer support groups. (See under Useful Addresses at the end of this book.)

Questions and exercises

(1) The primary nurse is aware that a long-term detained patient does not have an identified nearest relative and no visitors come to see him. She considers that there would be advantages if one

were to be appointed. What action could be taken and what procedure should be followed?

(2) Of the following relatives, who would be defined as the nearest? (a) father; (b) son of 16 years; (c) half-brother; (d) separated spouse; and (e) aunt.

(3) The patient had lived in a residential home for over seven years before being compulsorily admitted to a psychiatric hospital. She has no known relatives. Could the person who shared her two-bedded room at the residential home and was a friend be defined as the nearest relative?

(4) The mother and nearest relative of a detained patient is herself admitted to psychiatric hospital, she is not prepared to give up the position of nearest relative. A sister of the patient is prepared to act. What action could be taken?

(5) An informal patient does not have any statutory friend comparable to the nearest relative. Do you think that this is a gap which should be filled and if so how?

Chapter 8   Consent to treatment

General Principles

Every adult mentally competent person has a right to give or withhold consent to treatment unless exceptional circumstances justify an exception to this principle. In the absence of such justification a person who is treated without his consent can bring an action for trespass to the person. This is a civil action where harm does not need to be proved. The actual touching is known as 'a battery'; the apprehension that there will be an unlawful touching is known as 'an assault'.

The exceptional circumstances referred to above where an action would otherwise be a trespass to the person include:

- arrest by citizen or policeman under the Police and Criminal Evidence Act 1984 (this is not further discussed in this book);
- treatment given without consent under Part IV of the Mental Health Act 1983; and
- treatment given under the power at common law recognized by the House of Lords in the case of *F* v. *West Berkshire Health Authority* (1989) (see below and Glossary) where it was held that a professional who acted in the best interests of a person unable to give consent and who followed the reasonable standard of care would not be acting unlawfully.

Reference should be made to Chapter 15 of the Code of Practice. The general principles of consent and capacity are given in paragraphs 15.8 to 15.24.

One of the most significant of the changes introduced by the Act of 1983 was the control over the circumstances in which detained patients could be given treatment without their consent. Part IV of the Act sets out the conditions for giving treatment to detained patients. Important aspects concerning treatment are summarized under parts (1) to (5) of this chapter below. Part (2) covers treatments including those requiring consent and a second opinion under Part IV of the Act. This and part (3) on documentation and forms give vital information for nurses. Reference should also be made to Chapter 16 of the Code of Practice.

(1) Who is covered under Part IV of the Act?

Not all those patients under a section are covered by Part IV. Figure 8.1 sets out those short-term sections under which patients are **not** covered by the consent to treatment provisions.

Figure 8.1 Detained Patients *outside* the provisions of Part IV of the Act.

- Patients under sections 4, 5(2), 5(4), 35, 135 and 136.
- Patients subject to the directions of the court under section 37(4) pending admission to hospital.
- Restricted patients conditionally discharged under section 42(2) or section 73 or section 74 and who have not been recalled to hospital.

(See Appendix I(A) for section details.)

What applies to patients outside Part IV?

The legal position of patients listed in Fig 8.1 in relation to consent to treatment is that no compulsory treatment can be given to these patients under the provisions of the Act. In a situation of **necessity** it would be possible to give treatment under the powers that exist at common law. These powers were discussed by the House of Lords in the case of *F* v. *West Berkshire Health Authority (1989)*. It is clear that they would justify action being taken in the case of a patient who lacked the capacity to give consent. Treatment could be given in the patient's best interests according to reasonable professional standards. (For further details of the common law powers see below.)

However, it is uncertain how far it would be legal to give treatment to anyone against his will where the patient under these short term sections is capable of decision. It is preferable if at all possible to wait until the patient is placed under a long term section.

(2) Treatment

Treatment is given a wide definition in section 145(1) of the Act: ' "Medical treatment" includes nursing, and also includes care, habilitation and rehabilitation under medical supervision'.

It is difficult to consider any treatment of the patient which does not come under this definition. It would also include psychological procedures and behavioural programmes. For the purpose of Part IV of the Act treatment for mental disorder is divided into the following categories:

- Surgical treatment involving the destruction of brain tissue, surgical implantation of hormones for the purpose of reducing male sex drive and other treatments which may be prescribed by the Secretary of State – section 57 applies.
- Electro-convulsive therapy (ECT) – section 58 applies.
- The first three months of medication given after the patient is detained – section 63 applies.
- Medication given after the first three months that that medication was first administered – section 58 applies.
- All other treatments – section 63 applies.
- Urgent treatments. In certain urgent situations, when section 57 and section 58 would normally apply, treatment can be given under section 62.

Treatment for physical disorders

Sections 57, 58 and 63 refer specifically to treatment for mental disorder. It has therefore been interpreted that these provisions of the Act do not apply to treatments which are for physical disorders.

The point is important since it raises the basic question as to whether physical treatment required as a direct result of the patient's mental disorder is covered by the provisions of the Act. Thus a patient admitted under section 3 in a very dishevelled state might refuse to have a much needed bath. Could he be compelled to have this under section 63 (see Appendix I(A) for precise wording) since it is 'medical treatment', which is defined to include 'care', recommended by a responsible medical officer (RMO) and given under his direction? Those who take the restricted view that the provisions only apply where the treatment is for mental disorder would argue that bathing is not covered under section 63 and could only be given, if at all, by common law powers. Others would argue that the cleaning of a patient is actually connected with help for his mental disorder since it is part of the rehabilitation/treatment process. These issues assume even more importance in the cases of those suffering from anorexia nervosa where the first requirement is often to feed that patient to prevent death by starvation.

Some assistance has now been provided by the case of *B* v. *Croydon Health Authority* (1994). In this case a patient suffering from a psychopathic disease was admitted under section 3. The Court of Appeal held that feeding by tube could be administered to her compulsorily under section 63, even though that was not the treatment which justified admission under section 3.

> 'Nursing and care concurrent with the core treatment or as a necessary prerequisite to such treatment or to prevent the patient from causing harm to himself or to alleviate the consequences of the disorder were all capable of being ancillary to a treatment calculated to alleviate or prevent a deterioration of the psychopathic disorder' (Lord Justice Hoffman)

A similar issue has arisen in relation to the administration of a new drug known as clozapine (clozaril). Because of the known side effects of this drug on leucocytes, blood must be monitored weekly for the first 18 weeks then fortnightly. The treatment must be withdrawn if the leucocyte count falls below a certain level. It has been held that, if this drug is given compulsorily to a detained patient on the basis of a second opinion doctor's recommendation (see below), the right to give the treatment compulsorily should also include the power to take a blood sample whenever required. Reference should be made to the Mental Health Act Commission Practice Note Number 1.

Urgent treatments – section 62

The circumstances in which urgent treatment can be given are set out in Figure 8.2. Section 62 does **not** apply to informal patients and only covers treatments which come under section 57 or section 58.

No statutory forms have been drawn up to be used in connection with section 62 but it is helpful if there are forms completed giving the circumstances where section 62 treatments have been applied and the nature of the treatment administered. An example of a possible form is given in Appendix II, Example C.

Brain surgery and surgical implantation of hormones – section 57

Section 57 governs the following treatments for mental disorder:

- brain surgery destroying brain tissue, and
- hormonal implants to control male sex drive.

The detailed provisions relating to these treatments are given in Appendix I(A). The section also applies to informal patients. They cannot therefore be given such treatment against their will and, even if they wish to have the treatment, they could be overruled if the second opinion doctor does not agree that the

Treatment	Prerequisite	Purpose
Any	Immediately necessary	To save life
Not irreversible*	Immediately necessary	To prevent serious deterioration
Not irreversible or hazardous*	Immediately necessary	To alleviate suffering
Not irreversible or hazardous*	Immediately necessary and represents minimum interference	To prevent patient from behaving violently or being a danger to himself or to others
Continuation of treatment	Immediately necessary	If discontinuance of a treatment plan would cause serious suffering to the patient

Note Definitions of 'irreversible' and 'hazardous' are given in section 62(3).

Figure 8.2 Urgent treatment – section 62.

treatment should proceed. The Secretary of State has the power to specify by regulation other forms of treatment to come under section 57, as he has done in the case of hormonal implants. However he has a statutory duty to consult with such bodies as appear to him to be concerned before he makes any such regulations under section 57.

The operation of section 57 has come under the scrutiny of the courts in a case where the Commissioners had refused to give approval to the treatment proceeding (*R* v. *Mental Health Act Commission, ex parte W* (1988)).

The nurse has an important role to play in the consultation process and this is discussed below in connection with section 58.

Electro-convulsive therapy (ECT) and medication after three months – section 58

Section 58 covers ECT and medication after the expiry of three months from the time that medication was first administered to a detained patient. Such treatments can only be given **either** with the consent of the patient **or** with the agreement of a second opinion doctor. The provisions of section 58 are given in Appendix I(A). It is important for the nurse to be aware of the three month period from initial medication and when it elapses since there will be a breach of the Act if section 58 is not implemented at the appropriate time. Hospitals should set up a system to check on the date that consent under section 58 becomes due. If the nurse is aware that this system is lacking she should take action to ensure it is established.

Under section 58(3) (see Appendix I(A)), it can be seen that the patients fall into two categories:

- those who have given a valid consent, and
- those who are incapable of giving consent or refuse to give consent.

It is essential that the nurse appreciates the difference, since those patients who have given consent can withdraw it at any time and treatment cannot then be given without a second opinion doctor (SOAD) being brought in (subject to the possibility of section 62 being applicable).

(3) Documentation regarding consent

Consent forms

Form 38 is completed when the patient has given consent. Form 39 is completed when the SOAD has seen the patient and considers that treatment should be given in the absence of consent (statutory forms are listed in Appendix II).

It is preferable if copies of the appropriate form are kept with the medicine cards since this will enable the nurse when she administers the drugs to understand the nature of the consent and to know what action should be taken if the patient refuses to take the prescribed medication.

If a Form 38 has been completed and the patient subsequently refuses medication, then the nurse does not have the legal right to compel the patient to take the medication. The doctor should be informed of the patient's refusal and, if appropriate, section 62 could be used for urgent treatment to be given compulsorily to the patient until a SOAD can be summoned to decide if compulsory treatment is appropriate.

The nurse should also be able to check that the medicines prescribed are within the dosages set out on either Form 38 or Form 39. This is particularly important where medicines given as required (PRN) are concerned since there is a danger that the PRN medication plus the prescribed drugs could exceed the dosages set out on Forms 38 or 39.

What if the nurse is not satisfied that Forms 38 or 39 are correct?

Errors on Forms 38 and 39 might include the following:

- Form 38 has not been signed by the responsible medical officer of the patient.
- Form 38 or 39 does not correspond with what has been written up on the prescription sheets:
  (a) there might be different drugs
  (b) the dosages prescribed might be higher than those written on Forms 38 or 39.
- The SOAD might not have included his name and address

In such circumstances the nurse should not administer the drug but seek urgent advice on the legality of the prescription and attempt to rectify the situation urgently. She may feel reluctant to cause problems, especially where the patient appears willing to take whatever medication is offered. However, it is her personal responsibility, for which she is professionally accountable, to ensure that the law is complied with in the administration of the treatment and she should make every effort to ensure that both the letter and the spirit of the law is followed.

Hospital consent forms

Hospitals often have their own consent forms whether for ECT or medication or both. However this does not remove the need to ensure that Form 38 or 39 is completed in respect of ECT and/or medication. Forms 38 or 39 constitute the legal authority for giving treatment to a detained patient under section 58. The form should be filled in with a maximum number of applications of ECT so that the patient could be given up to that number but no more without bringing in a SOAD again (Form 39), or review by the RMO and fresh consent by the patient (Form 38). The form should give details of the dosage to be given of any medication, usually in relation to the maximum levels recommended in the British National Formulary.

PRN policy

The nurse should ensure that there is in existence a policy which covers the writing up and administration of PRN medication. The prescription should set out not only the dose and the route of administration but also the intervals and the maximum which can be given in any 24 hour period, together with the date when the prescription should be reviewed.

Form 39 and the second opinion appointed doctor

The SOAD (see below) must consult two persons who have been professionally concerned with the patient's medical treatment. One must be a nurse; the other must be neither a nurse nor a registered medical practitioner.

In consulting the nurse and other professionals under section 57 and 58, the doctor simply has to record the names and professions of those he has consulted and the date. However there is considerable advantage if the nurse also records in her notes the fact of the consultation and the views she expressed and the reasons behind those views. This means that if there is any subsequent debate over the treatment the nurse has a comprehensive record of the circumstances.

The opportunity for the nurse to be involved in this discussion is significant. She is likely to have an extensive day to day knowledge of the patient. She should know the patient's own preferences and it is important that the nurse is prepared to put her viewpoint succinctly and logically to the doctor. Training in this role is strongly recommended. It also means that the nurse should have a good understanding of the various drugs and their alternatives and the advantages and disadvantages of ECT.

(4) Decisions on treatment

The independent medical practitioner

The independent medical practitioner has to be appointed by the Secretary of State who has delegated this task to the Mental Health Act Commission (MHAC) which arranges for the doctors to be sent to the hospitals following a request under section 57 or 58 and also arranges training schemes for these doctors who are known as second opinion appointed doctors (SOADs). The distinction should be drawn between the practice of referring to a second opinion on the patient's treatment and diagnosis by the patient's general practitioner or consultant. A SOAD under the Act is statutorily required to see the patient before compulsory treatment can be given in certain specified circumstances (see paragraphs 16.9 and 16.26 to 16.32 of the Code of Practice).

Dispute between the SOAD and the RMO

If the SOAD always agrees with the patient's own doctor there would be no point in having the second opinion system. It would simply be a rubber stamping exercise. There are occasions when the SOAD does not support the recommendations of the patient's own doctor. In such a case it is anticipated that they will together discuss the treatment and eventually agree on an alternative course of treatment. If it is impossible to secure agreement between the RMO and the SOAD, a request could be made to the MHAC for another SOAD to be appointed. The RMO remains clinically responsible for the care of the patient.

(5) Other points on treatment

Treatment plans

The consent given under section 57 and 58 can relate to a treatment plan by which the patient can be given one or more of the forms of treatment to which the section applies (section 59). If the patient has given his consent to any of the treatments he can withdraw this consent at any time. If appropriate the provisions of section 62 could then be used to give treatment without consent (see section 60).

Review of treatment – section 61

If the patient is being given treatment under section 57 or is subject to the second opinion system under section 58(3)(b), each time there is a report by the RMO recommending renewal of the patient's section a report on the treatment and the patient's condition must be given by the RMO to the Secretary of State. The Secretary of State has delegated this duty of receiving reports and reviewing the matter to the MHAC. A Mental Health Act Commission Form (MHAC 1) has to be completed (listed in Appendix II). There is similar provision for reports to be furnished on patients who are subject to a restriction order or a restriction direction or at any time the Secretary of State or the MHAC requests one.

Treatment not requiring consent

Section 63 makes provision for treatment not falling under sections 57 or 58. The conditions of section 63 are very wide (see Appendix I(A)) and mean that essentially any treatment **not** specified under Sections 57 or 58 can be given without the consent of the patient.

There is concern that the scope of section 63 is too wide. Certain psychological treatments could be given without the consent of the patient. There is a suggestion that such treatments should be subject to section 58 controls and should be specified by the Secretary of State as coming under Section 58. There is also debate as to whether section 63 could be used to cover seclusion of the patient. In the case *B* v. *Croydon Health Authority* (1994) (see above) it was held that feeding by tube could come under section 63.

Treatment for physical disorders

In the case of *Re C (adult: refusal of medical treatment)* (1994), a Broadmoor patient succeeded in obtaining an injunction against the hospital restraining it from carrying out an amputation without his express written consent. It was held that even though he suffered from paranoid schizophrenia the evidence failed to show that he lacked sufficient understanding of the nature, purpose and effect of the proposed treatment (which the doctors believed to be necessary to save his life), but instead showed that he had understood and retained the relevant treatment information, believed it and had arrived at a clear choice. The presumption in favour of his right to self-determination had not been displaced.

Informal patients

Part IV gives the protection of the Act to informal patients in respect of treatments for mental disorder requiring surgery involving the loss of brain tissue and also for hormonal implants by surgery to reduce male sex drive. These treatments cannot be carried out on an informal patient unless the conditions of section 57 are complied with (see Appendix I(A) for wording).

Apart from that provision there are no statutory provisions regulating the giving of consent by the non-detained patient. This also applies to those patients on short-term sections, who are outside the provisions of Part IV (see Figure 8.1).

Informal patients constitute by far the greater number of patients under the care of nurses. Many informal patients will be incapable of giving a valid consent. There is at present no system of proxy decision making by which a nominated person would have the power to give consent on their behalf. The possibility of setting up such a system is under active consideration by the Law Commission (see *Decision Making and the Mentally Incapacitated Adult*, Papers No. 119, 128, 129 and 130). The Law Commission in its Report No. 231 (see Appendix I(D)) has recommended statutory provision for decision making on behalf of the mentally incapacitated adult.

Where the patient is incapable of giving a valid consent, professionals would act lawfully if they acted in the best interests of the patient and followed the accepted approved professional practice. This was the law laid down by the House of Lords in *F* v. *West Berkshire Health Authority* (1989) (see Glossary). The ruling given in this case would also apply to the work of a nurse.

Day to day care however could be carried out by the nurse without the consent of the patient provided that it was in the best interests of the patient. In this area the relatives have no right in law to give or withhold consent. However it would obviously be good practice to ensure that they were consulted and had an input into the discussions over what was in the best interests of the patient.

The nurse should remember that in such cases the patient is outside of the protection provided by the Act for the detained patient. She should therefore ensure that the patient is no worse off as a result of that fact. If she has serious concerns over the best interests of the patient and the extent to which the patient is adequately protected she might draw the doctor's attention to the possibility of the patient being detained under a section. Unfortunately incompetent patients who do not protest but accept treatment passively are rarely sectioned and therefore do not receive the protection of the statutory provisions.

The situation of a patient's refusal to consent to essential treatment was considered by the court in the case of *Re T* (1992) (see Glossary). In this case the Court of Appeal emphasized the patient's right to give or withhold consent to treatment, but the professional had a duty to check that the refusal was valid, which, in the particular circumstances of this case, it was not.

Patients who are minors

Minors have the right to consent to treatment under the Family Law Reform Act 1969 when they are 16 years and over. Treatment includes diagnostic procedures and an anaesthetic. Minors who are younger than that can also consent to treatment if they have the maturity to understand what is involved and to give a valid consent, a level of competence that was defined by the House of Lords in the case of *Gillick* v. *West Norfolk and Wisbech Area Health Authority* (1985).

However in the case of *Re W (a minor) (medical treatment)* (1992) the Court of Appeal endorsed the decision of the High Court judge who gave approval to the overruling of the wishes of a girl of 16 years who suffered from anorexia nervosa and who refused treatment. She was not a detained patient and the provisions of the Mental Health Act 1983 were not therefore relevant. The Court of Appeal stated that:

> 'There could be no doubt that the court had power to override the refusal of a minor, whether over 16 or under 16 and Gillick competent.'

The Children's Act 1989, which places emphasis on the child agreeing to medical treatment and future provision, did not prevent this right of the court applying.

Preceding consent to treatment

What if a patient when not mentally disordered signed an agreement that treatment could be given to him without his consent when he became mentally disordered? Would such a document be valid in law?

The answer is probably 'no' although such a statement has not yet been tested in a court of law. The reason is that the person who signed such a statement and who was compelled to undergo treatment against his will when he became mentally disordered would lose the protection that Part IV of the Act gives to detained patients. There need be no SOAD nor consultation with other professionals. Nor can it be certain that the conditions which existed when the patient signed the form still exist. The danger is that the patient, having been forced when mentally disordered to undergo treatment, might protest after he has recovered that the signature did not bind him and in those circumstances he could sue for trespass to the person. The professionals who cared for him would then be faced with defending a court action and justifying their actions on the basis of a document whose validity is now disputed by the patient. They would be in a far stronger position if the patient were detained and the provisions of Part IV of the Act were therefore followed or if they could rely on the doctrine of necessity and acting in the best interests of the patient under the ruling in *F* v. *West Berkshire Area Health Authority* (1989).

Preceding refusal of treatment

The use of 'living wills' or 'advance directives' is being reviewed by the Law Commission as part of its consideration of decision making by the mentally incompetent adult. It is essential that such pre-directives are also considered in the context of the care of the mentally disordered.

The Select Committee of the House of Lords on Medical Ethics has supported the Law Commission's recommendation on advance refusal of treatment and suggests a Code of Practice should be drawn up (Select Committee of House of Lords on Medical Ethics, *Report of Session 1993/94*). Clause 9 of the Mental Incapacity Bill drafted by the Law Commission in its Report No. 231 enables a person of 18 years or more to give 'an advance refusal of treatment' (see Appendix I(D)).

Questions and exercises

(1) An extremely mentally disordered patient who agreed to be admitted as an informal patient is refusing any treatment. What action, if any should the nurse take?

(2) A patient who has been detained for four months on section 3 agrees to a treatment plan for medication. Two weeks later he changes his mind. What action, if any, should the nurse take and what is the legal situation?

(3) How are the following treatments covered by the statutory provisions in the case of a patient detained under Section 2? (a) ECT; (b) clozapine; (c) aversion therapy; (d) brain surgery; and (e) time out.

(4) The RMO has signed Form 38 in respect of 12 treatments for ECT. After five treatments the patient refuses to give consent. The RMO considers it would be dangerous for the patient if ECT were stopped at this time. What action can be taken in law?

(5) The SOAD consults with you in the treatment to be given to a patient who is refusing to consent. What relevant circumstances do you consider should be brought to his attention and what records would you keep of your discussions?

Chapter 9   Appeals against detention

Depriving individuals of their liberty is one of the greatest invasions of their rights. It is essential that there should be a clear appeal mechanism which is speedily and easily enforceable. Figure 9.1 sets out the main forms of appeal open to those detained under the Mental Health Act (1983).

- Appeal to a Mental Health Review Tribunal (MHRT) as set out in Part V of the Act and discussed in this chapter
- An appeal to the Managers under section 23
- An order for discharge by the nearest relative
- A writ of *habeas corpus*
- An action for false imprisonment

Figure 9.1 Appeals against or challenges to detention.

Most of this chapter is concerned with appeals to the MHRT, which is the most important way of challenging the detention of the patient.

Applications and referrals to the Mental Health Review Tribunals

Since 1983 there is a statutory duty on the managers to refer a detained patient to the MHRT if neither he nor his nearest relative has applied for review within defined time limits, or if he has applied and the application has been withdrawn.

The circumstances as to when there can be an application to the MHRT, by whom it can be made and at what time are somewhat complex (section 66). A simplification of section 66 is set out in Figure 9.2. It is assumed that section 3 follows on from section 2.

Referral by managers

The managers must automatically refer the patient to an MHRT (if he has failed to apply himself, or if the application has been withdrawn) within the first six months of detention and every

Authority for detention	Months from admission	The relevant period (Timing)
Section 2	1	Within 14 days from admission
Section 3	2–7	Between 2nd and 7th month from admission to Section
Section 3	8–13	If renewal of Section
Section 3	13–24	If renewal for 12 months
Section 3	25–36	If renewal for 12 months
Section 3	37–48	If renewal for 12 months

Figure 9.2 Applications to an MHRT by patient

three years thereafter. Thus apathy, ignorance or other reasons should not result in the patient not coming before a hearing for many years. The timings and conditions for patients under various sections are given in Figure 9.3.

Authority for detention	Timing	Conditions
Section 3	After the first six months and after three years*	If no application is heard by MHRT, Managers must refer
Section 37	After second six months – then if no hearing after three years*	If no application is heard by MHRT, Managers must refer
Section 41	If no hearing within previous three years	Referral by Home Secretary**

Notes *Annually for patients under 16 years.
**In addition the Home Secretary may refer at any time.

Figure 9.3 Automatic referral to an MHRT by managers.

Application to an MHRT by nearest relative

There are certain circumstances under which the nearest relative can make application to an MHRT. The situation is summarized in Figure 9.4.

Authority for detention	Timing	Conditions
Sections 4, 5(2) and (4)	—	No right of application
Section 3	Within 28 days	After being informed that RMO report bars discharge of patient
Section 37	Within second six months then annually	For patients under hospital and guardianship orders
Sections 37 and 41	—	No right of application by nearest relative for those under restriction orders
Section 16	Within 28 days	After reclassification of patient's mental disorder

Figure 9.4 Application to an MHRT by nearest relative.

Important aspects of the Mental Health Review Tribunal system

Figure 9.5 lists important aspects of appeal to an MHRT which are discussed below.

(a) Constitution of the MHRT
(b) Powers
(c) Procedure pre-hearing and hearing
(d) Role of the nurse
(e) Financial aid
(f) Legal representation
(g) Appeals against the decisions
(h) Forms and official documentation
(i) Confidentiality
(j) Withdrawal of applications

Figure 9.5 Important aspects of appeal to an MHRT.

(a) Constitution of the MHRT

Schedule 2 of the Act sets out the composition of an MHRT and additional regulations are laid down by the Mental Health Review Tribunal Rules 1983 (SI 1983 No. 942). The panel on the tribunal has legal members, medical members and other members with knowledge of administration, social services or other suitable qualifications.

Full details of the rules governing MHRTs can be found in Part 2 of Richard Jones' *Mental Health Act Manual.*

(b) Powers

The MHRT has the right to discharge patients from certain sections if the specified conditions are met. More detail is given below. In this context it is crucial to bear in mind that discharge from a section does not mean discharge from the hospital or from care (see Chapter 4 part (1)).

The MHRT **must** discharge a patient detained under section 2 if satisfied that the conditions set out in Figure 9.6 are present.

Figure 9.6
Circumstances in which a section 2 patient should be discharged by the MHRT – section 72(1)(a) of the Act.

The MHRT **must** discharge **if** they are satisfied:

(1) that the patient is not then suffering from mental disorder or from mental disorder of a nature or degree which warrants his detention in a hospital for assessment (or for assessment followed by medical treatment) for at least a limited period; or

(2) that such detention is not justified in the interests of the patient's own health or safety or with a view to the protection of other persons.

For patients **other than** those detained under section 2, the tribunal **must** discharge the patient if the circumstances set out in Figure 9.7 exist.

For patients (other than those under Section 2), where the

Figure 9.7
Circumstances in which detained patients other than those on section 2 must be discharged by the MHRT – section 72(1)(b) of the Act.

The MHRT **must** discharge **if** they are satisfied:

(1) that the patient is not then suffering from mental illness, psychopathic disorder, severe mental impairment or mental impairment or from any of those forms of disorder of a nature or degree which makes it appropriate for him to be liable to be detained in a hospital for medical treatment; or

(2) that it is not necessary for the health or safety of the patient or for the protection of other persons that he should receive such treatment; or

(3) that the patient, if released, would not be likely to act in a manner dangerous to other persons or to himself (in cases where the RMO has barred discharge by the nearest relative).

provisions of Figure 9.7 are **not** satisfied so that the tribunal does not **have** to discharge the patient, it can use discretionary powers to discharge, having regard to the matters listed in Figure 9.8 (section 72(2)).

Figure 9.8 Factors the MHRT must consider where it is not bound to discharge the patient under Figure 9.7 above.

> The MHRT must consider:
>
> (1) the likelihood of medical treatment alleviating or preventing a deterioration of the patient's condition; and
>
> (2) in the case of a patient suffering from mental illness or severe mental impairment, the likelihood of the patient, if discharged, being able to care for himself, to obtain the care he needs or to guard himself against serious exploitation.

The tribunal can direct the patient to be discharged on a future date which it specifies (section 72(3) of the Act).

If the tribunal does **not** direct the discharge of the patient, it may:

(a) with a view to facilitating his discharge on a future date, recommend that he be granted leave of absence or be transferred to another hospital or into guardianship and give further consideration if the recommendation is not complied with (section 72(3) of the Act); or

(b) if satisfied that the patient is suffering from a form of mental disorder other than the form specified in the application, order or direction relating to him, rule that these be amended (section 72(5) of the Act).

Further provision exists for patients under a restriction order (see Chapter 5).

(c) Procedure pre-hearing

An application must be made in writing to the MHRT. Applications may be made by letter or on an appropriate form. Examples of Form 1 (which applies to patients detained under section 2) and Form 2 (which applies to patients detained under sections 3, 37, 47 or 48, or treated as if detained under one of those sections) can be found in Appendix II (Examples D and E).

The patient should be given the relevant application form by the hospital staff and advised of his rights to have legal representation and given assistance in contacting a solicitor (should he so wish) and in meeting with one. He should be assisted in the completion of the application form. Should he wish to have an independent medical examination this should be facilitated.

Nearest relatives are also notified of their rights to attend the tribunal hearing and to be accompanied by any other person. They can also authorize a representative such as a solicitor to act for them.

The nearest relative can write to the tribunal in advance of the date of the hearing with information or comments about the patient, indicating which parts they would not wish to be disclosed to the patient.

The hearing

Detailed rules are set out in the Mental Health Review Tribunal Rules 1983 (SI 1983 No. 942). The procedure is flexible so that the review can be held in a manner which is most suitable for the patient. The President of the Tribunal will explain how the case is to be conducted. The location will also take into account the patient's needs. The emphasis should be on informality, so that the patient and others not used to such occasions will not be intimidated.

Reports will have been provided by the RMO in charge of the care of the patient and also by the social worker. In addition the nurse may be asked to prepare a report. Any submissions in writing should be shown to the patient unless the writer considers that the disclosure to the patient would adversely affect the health or welfare of the patient or others in which case the reasons for believing that its disclosure would have that effect should be stated (Tribunal Rules, paragraph 32.2).

(d) Role of nurse

The nurse must ensure the following:

- that the patient has the appropriate knowledge about the application and an application form,
- that arrangements are being made for him to receive legal (or other) representation should he so wish,
- that, if requested, she prepares a report for the hearing, deciding which parts (if any) have to be excluded from disclosure to the patient, and
- that she is prepared to give evidence before the tribunal should this be requested.

For the last two points, the nurse should study carefully the requirements laid out in Figures 9.6, 9.7 and 9.8 and include relevant observations in her report.

(e) Financial aid

This is available under the legal aid advice and assistance scheme.

(f) Legal representation

Many more patients are now seeking legal representation because the right to obtain legal aid has been introduced.

(g) Appeals against the tribunal's decision

An appeal can be made to the High Court against a decision of the MHRT on a point of law, or where no reasonable tribunal would have come to that decision on the evidence before them. When requested to do so by the High Court, Section 78(8) requires an MHRT to state any question of law which may arise before them in the form of a special case for determination by the High Court.

In addition an application can be made for judicial review by the High Court of the proceedings of the tribunal. This power can be used if, for example, there is a suggestion that the rules of natural justice were not followed, for example the patient did not have an opportunity to put forward his case, or have it put forward on his behalf, or if there was bias on the part of the tribunal.

(h) Forms and official documentation

There is no prescribed form for the application, but it must be in writing. For convenience, application forms are available from the tribunal offices (See Appendix II, Examples D and E). Under Rule 32, the responsible managers must provide the tribunal with copies of the admission papers and the information set out in Part A, Schedule 1 to the Rules.

(i) Confidentiality

The hearing is not usually a public hearing and the press cannot insist on attending. Matters therein are kept confidential. If the patient wishes, however, the hearing can be held in public.

(j) Withdrawal of application

Should a patient withdraw an application for a hearing the hearing will not usually proceed, unless the tribunal decides it should proceed under Rule 19. However the managers have a duty to refer to a tribunal a patient who has not applied or who has withdrawn an application (see Figure 9.3).

Appeals to the managers

The detained patient, as well as having a right to apply to an MHRT, can also apply to the managers for discharge from the section. In contrast to the application to an MHRT, there are no specific timings for making such an application and there is no specified statutory procedure to be followed.

The identity of the managers

The definition of who the managers are for the purposes of appeal under section 23 is stipulated in section 23(4) which states that the powers under section 23 may be exercised by any three or more of the members of the Health Authority or body authorized by it or by a committee or sub-committee of that authority or body which has been authorized by them in that behalf.

In the newly formed NHS Trusts additional members have been appointed by the Authority for the purposes of carrying out duties under the Mental Health Act 1983 and these therefore supplement the few non-executive members in such tasks. The legality of this was questioned, and amending legislation was introduced in 1994 so that non-executive directors could be supplemented to hear an appeal. Executive directors or officers of the NHS Trusts cannot hear appeals.

Mental Health Act Managers cannot delegate the power to discharge patients. All other statutory duties placed on the managers can be delegated (see Chapter 19).

The legality of the detention

Under section 6(2), where the patient is admitted within the appropriate period to hospital, the application shall be sufficient authority for the managers to detain the patient in hospital in accordance with the provisions. Forms 14 and 15 are completed by the managers to give evidence of receipt of the medical recommendations and the application, and to record the time and date of admission of the patient. The Mental Health Act Managers can delegate this task to officers, usually to Mental Health Act Administrators.

Managers' obligation to review

The managers can review the detention of a patient at any time and **must** review the detention:

- on a request from the patient,
- if the RMO provides a report under section 20 for the renewal of detention, or
- if the RMO bars the nearest relative's discharge application.

The managers cannot delegate this task but their numbers can be supplemented as above. Three or more managers must hear the review.

There should be a hearing procedure which covers the pre-review stages, the review itself and the steps to be followed post-review. There are no statutory guidelines for undertaking the review and hearings vary according to the degree of formality which is followed. The book *Hearing Patients' Appeals against continued compulsory detention* (Williamson, 1991) offers guidance for managers. The review could be challenged by the patient who might seek a judicial review before the High Court if the principles of natural justice have not been followed. The Code of Practice gives a list of considerations which should be taken into account in the conduct of the review (see Code of Practice paragraphs 22.1 to 22.6).

Other routes for appeal

Order for discharge by the nearest relative

This is a matter subject to fuller discussion in Chapter 7.

Application for *habeas corpus*

At present a writ for *habeas corpus* can be issued when a case of false imprisonment is alleged to be taking place. It is dealt with urgently. Literally it calls upon the defendant to produce the body which he has. This action could be used by informal patients who are kept in seclusion or prevented from leaving a hospital, home or other institution without lawful justification. It can also be used on behalf of a detained patient who alleges that his detention is illegal.

Action for false imprisonment

This action is a civil action and a variant of the action for trespass to the person. It can be brought to obtain compensation in the civil courts where it is alleged that a person has been falsely detained without lawful justification. It could therefore be used by any informal patient who claims that he was secluded or unjustifiably prevented from leaving the hospital. No harm has to be established other than the loss of liberty. It must be shown that the imprisonment was complete and that there was no reasonable form of escape.

Questions and exercises

(1) You are approached by a patient detained under section 2 who wishes to apply to an MHRT. What are his rights:

    (a)   if he has been detained for 7 days, or

    (b)   if he has been detained for 21 days?

What other forms of appeal are open to him?

(2)   A patient on your ward has been detained for over three years and you are not aware that he has ever been referred to an MHRT. What action would you take?

(3)   You are the primary nurse for a patient who is due to appear before an MHRT and who has asked you if you would accompany her as a representative/friend? What action would you take? If you agreed to attend, what preparations would you make for the hearing?

(4)   You have been asked to prepare a written report for an MHRT hearing. What headings would you use and how would you set about it?

(5)   What differences are there between a hearing before an MHRT and a hearing before the managers?

Chapter 10 Leave with consent under section 17

Who can authorize leave?

The responsible medical officer (RMO) (who is the doctor or consultant in charge of the treatment of the patient), and **only** the RMO, may grant leave to be absent from hospital to any detained patient under section 17 (see Figure 10.1). He can place any conditions on such leave which he considers are necessary in the interests of the patient or for the protection of other persons (section 17(1)). Where a patient is under a restriction order or direction, the RMO can only grant leave of absence with the consent of the Home Secretary (see below). The wording of section 17 is given in Appendix I(A).

---

(1) The RMO may grant
(2) to any patient detained under the Act
(3) leave to be absent from the hospital
(4) subject to the conditions (if any) considered by the RMO necessary
   ● in the interests of the patient, or
   ● for the protection of other persons.

Figure 10.1 Grant of leave of absence – section 17(1).

It is thus possible for the patient as part of the long-term treatment plan to have time away from the original place of detention. The decision to grant leave should be part of a multi-disciplinary discussion in which all those professionals who would be involved in the discussion of the after-care programmes should have an input. Leave should be part of the long-term plans which eventually lead to discharge. However section 17 should not be used in place of discharge if that is more appropriate. In addition the relatives/carers and the patient himself should also be involved in the discussions.

The restricted patient

The patient who is under restriction, such as patients under section 41 (see Chapter 5), can only be granted leave if the Home Office gives consent. The RMO would provide the Home Office with all the relevant details concerning the type of leave which is recommended, the location, the length proposed and would also give full details of the patient's present condition and the reasons why leave of absence is being proposed. There have been considerable delays in obtaining decisions from the Home Office on requests for section 17 leave and it is important not to build up the patient's hopes too soon since the wait can be very frustrating. The nurse should ensure that she is aware of the actual position.

For how long?

Leave can be granted indefinitely or on specific occasions or for any specified period. Further leave can be given (section 17(2)). The length of the leave cannot exceed the expiry of the order for detention or six months whichever is the earlier (see Chapter 11).

The Mental Health (Patients in the Community) Act 1995 includes a section amending section 17 to enable leave to be as long as twelve months.

Where can the patient go?

The RMO could direct that the patient should remain in custody whilst on leave. The patient could therefore make an escorted visit to another place. The provision also enables the patient to be kept in another hospital. Advantage is often taken of this provision to enable a detained patient to spend time in another hospital of reduced security as preparation for ultimate discharge. Special Hospitals sometimes make use of section 17 leave to enable a patient to stay in a regional secure unit as part of the rehabilitative process. It is also possible for the patient to stay in a hostel or similar half-way accommodation. The advantage is that the RMO still remains responsible for the patient who can, if necessary, be returned to the original hospital under the provisions discussed in Chapter 11.

The patient could also be given section 17 leave to stay in a nursing home which need not be registered to take detained patients. The choice of accommodation is at the discretion of the RMO.

Legal responsibilities

Whilst the decision to allow the patient to have leave of absence should be part of a multi-disciplinary decision-making team, the RMO alone has the statutory responsibility of granting it. He could be liable for any negligence in granting leave of absence if the patient harms himself or another person whilst on section 17 leave.

However, it is essential that the nursing staff bring to the attention of the RMO any significant change in the patient's condition which might be a factor against section 17 leave being granted. If a patient whilst on Section 17 leave causes harm to himself or another person various legal issues arise. If it can be established that the RMO was acting contrary to the practice which would have been adopted by an RMO following the accepted approved practice, and if this failure caused reasonably foreseeable harm, then the doctor could be held personally liable and his employer vicariously liable. If, however, it were established that the nurse had failed to inform the doctor of a significant change in the patient's condition, and that had the doctor known of this he would have refused to grant leave, then the nurse could become liable, and again the employer vicariously liable for her negligence.

Recording leave of absence

The report of inquiry chaired by Sir Louis Blom-Cooper into the death of an occupational therapist killed by a detained patient at the Edith Morgan Unit in Torbay (*Falling Shadows*, 1995) emphasized the importance of the RMO deciding if leave should be granted under section 17, and the necessity of ensuring that there is a clear policy in place and records kept of the decision by the RMO (see also Code of Practice, paragraphs 20.1 to 20.9).

Section 17 itself does not require that the grant of section 17 leave shall be in writing. However it is essential to set up a clear system where the decisions on leave under section 17 are recorded. It does not necessarily mean that the doctor has to approve each and every occasion on which the patient leaves the hospital. He might agree to a plan whereby the patient is given one night's leave of absence at his home every other week and daily visits to the local shops. It should be clear from the records what leave is escorted and what leave is unescorted. Clearly there should also be a system of recording information given to the relatives. Reference should be made to the Code of Practice paragraphs 20.1 to 20.10. A suggested form for section 17 leave can be found in Appendix II (Example F).

Medication whilst on section 17 leave

A patient on section 17 leave would still remain liable to the consent to treatment provisions under Part IV of the Act unless he is on one of the excluded sections (see Chapter 8). Treatment cannot be given compulsorily in the community, and refusal by a patient to take necessary medication would be a contra-indication to section 17 leave being granted if treatment during that time was required in the patient's best interests. If during the leave of absence the three months of medication under section 63 expires and section 58 comes into effect, a Form 38 or 39 must be completed. The fact that the patient is on section 17 leave does not eliminate that necessity.

Recalling the patient

The patient is subject to recall while on section 17 leave which is a matter covered in Chapter 11.

Questions and exercises

(1a) The RMO tells a detained patient he can go back home to his father's house and collect more clothes. No-one informed the father who came to the ward and finds the patient is missing. The patient is later found dead at home. What steps could be taken to prevent such an occurrence?

(1b) What is the liability of the RMO? What is the liability of the nurse if it is established that she knew the patient's condition had deteriorated when leave had been granted but before he left the hospital?

(2) How should consent to section 17 leave be recorded?

(3) How do you record which patients are on section 17 leave? Is it necessary for the RMO to give consent to every single exodus from the hospital? Does a vacant bed have to be kept for every patient who is on section 17 leave?

Chapter 11 Returning the patient to hospital

This chapter looks at the circumstances in which a patient can lawfully be returned to the hospital. The following circumstances will be discussed:

- Recalling the patient from section 17 leave.
- Recalling patients who have taken leave without consent (liable to be detained under the Mental Health Act 1983).
- Patients under guardianship.
- Informal patients.

Details for patients in these different circumstances are given below.

Patients given leave of absence under section 17

Sub-section (4) of section 17 enables the leave of absence to be revoked and the patient recalled to hospital. Figure 11.1 sets out the requirements.

Leave of absence can be **revoked** and the patient **recalled** to the hospital if:

(a) it appears to the **responsible medical officer** (RMO)
(b) that it is **necessary** to do so in the interests of the patient's health or safety or for the protection of other persons, and
(c) **notice in writing** is given by the RMO
(d) to the **patient** or to the **person** for the time being **in charge of the patient.**

Figure 11.1   Recalling the patient from section 17 leave.

The powers in Figure 11.1 are **not** available in the following circumstances:

- if the patient has ceased to be liable to be detained,
- if he has had six months continuous leave, unless he is absent without leave at the end of that period, or
- if he is a restricted patient.

The patient cannot be recalled from section 17 leave in order to renew the section. This was the decision made in the case of *R v. Hallstrom, ex parte W* and *R v. Gardner, ex parte L* (1985) (see Glossary).

If the patient refuses to respond to a notice under section 17(4) he can be brought back under the provisions of section 18 (see below).

Patients liable to be detained under the Act

If a detained patient absents himself **without** leave being given under Section 17, he can be taken into custody and returned to the hospital or place of guardianship under section 18.

This provision also covers those patients who fail to return to the hospital after section 17 leave expires or is revoked, or who absent themselves without permission from any place where they are required to reside.

Who can retake the patient?

- Any approved social worker.
- Any officer on the staff of the hospital.
- Any constable.
- Any person authorized in writing by the hospital manager.

Are there exceptions to these powers?

Section 18 retaking provisions do not apply:

(a) after the expiration of six months beginning with the first day of absence without leave*, or

(b) if the patient is liable to be detained under sections 2(4), 4(4), 5(2) or 5(4) and the period of detention has expired.

*Note The Mental Health (Patients in the Community) Act 1995 contains a section extending this period; previously the patient absent without leave could only be retaken up to 28 days after the absconsion began.

If the patient is returned within the six months set out above but only one week or less of the detention is left, then section 21(1) applies and the length of the detention period is extended by a week to enable the RMO to make a report to renew the section under section 20. The patient remains liable to be detained during the six months, even though the authority for his detention would have expired during that period.

The right of the patient to remain at liberty if he had been absent without leave for 28 days was removed by the Mental Health (Patients in the Community) Act 1995.

What if the patient takes refuge in a house?

Can section 18 powers be used to retake the patient in such circumstances? The answer is that unless the occupier of the house permits the entry of the person who is to retake the patient under section 18, there are no powers of entry granted by that section. In such a case it would be necessary to obtain a warrant to enter and search for a person liable to be detained under section 135(2). The requirements are set out in Figure 11.2.

A warrant authorizing any constable, who **may** be accompanied by

(a)   a registered medical practitioner, and/or
(b)   any person authorized by the Act to take or retake the patient

to enter premise if need be by force and remove a patient may be issued by a justice of the peace if:

(a)   a **constable** or other **person authorized** under the Act has given **information on oath**
(b)   that
   • there is **reasonable cause** to believe that the patient is to be found on premises within the jurisdiction of the justice; and
   • that admission to the premises **has been refused** or that a refusal of such admission is apprehended.

Figure 11.2   Warrant to enter premises to retake a patient – section 135(2).

*Note   There is a distinction in the requirement that the constable be accompanied between this section 135(2) and section 135(1) (see Figure 12.1).

Patients under guardianship

Guardianship is discussed in Chapter 15, but the provision for returning the patient to the specified place is considered here for completeness.

Section 18 also applies to patients subject to guardianship and if such a patient absents himself without leave of the guardian from the place at which he is required to reside, he may be taken into custody and returned to that place by:

• any officer on the staff of a local social services authority,
• any constable,
• any person authorized in writing by the guardian or a local social services authority.

Powers under the Police and Criminal Evidence Act 1984

The House of Lords has held in the case of *D'Souza* v. *The Director of Public Prosecutions* (1992) that section 17(1)(d) of the Police and Criminal Evidence Act 1984 authorizes a policeman to enter and search any premises for the purpose of recapturing a person who is unlawfully at large and whom he is pursuing. The detained patient who is without leave of absence is unlawfully at large.

Informal patients

Informal patients have the right to leave hospital whenever they wish. This could include the middle of the night or any time which is not normally socially acceptable. Unless the patient comes under the provisions of the circumstances set out in section 5(2) or 5(4), the patient cannot be detained and must be allowed to leave. Of course it might be appropriate to use all possible persuasion to encourage the patient to delay departure to a more acceptable time.

Procedures for action to be taken when a patient goes missing sometimes do not distinguish between the situation which exists in law when the patient is detained or liable to be detained and where the patient is informal. It thus happens that if an informal patient goes missing, the police are notified and there have been occasions where the police are known to have returned the patient to hospital. The basis of their power to do so in law is dubious, unless they are exercising the powers they have under section 136 (discussed in Chapter 13) or are using their powers of arrest given under public order legislation or the Police and Criminal Evidence Act 1984.

If a nurse is involved in such a situation and the police return an informal patient to the hospital against his will, she should clarify the grounds the police have used for the return of the informal patient.

But what if a nurse of the prescribed class is not available to detain the patient under section 5(4) (Nurse's Holding Power)?

If all the requirements for using section 5(4) exist but the senior nurse on duty is not of the prescribed class, what action can she take? If the patient is an in-patient who is receiving treatment for mental disorder and should not be allowed to leave in the interests of his own health or safety or for the protection of others then it might be possible to argue that the nurse, even though not of the prescribed category, should use the common law powers to act in an emergency to save life by delaying the patient's departure until a prescribed nurse can use section 5(4).

The House of Lords in the case of *Black* v. *Forsey* (1988) which was on the Mental Health (Scotland) Act 1984, recognized the right at common law for a private individual to detain an informal patient in a situation of necessity, where the patient is of unsound mind or a danger to himself or others.

The legality of this has not been tested in relation to the Mental Health Act 1983 (applicable to England and Wales) but the use of common law powers in the best interests of the patient would probably be justifiable under the ruling in *F* v. *West Berkshire Health Authority* (1989). However it could only justify a temporary detention. As soon as possible a nurse of the prescribed class or the registered medical practitioner (who ever can arrive first) should be summoned to consider detention under section 5(4) or section 5(2) respectively. There should be a locally drawn up procedure to advise staff on the action to be taken. If there is a risk that section 5(4) powers might be needed, there should be a nurse of the prescribed class on duty on the ward at all times.

Procedure for patients taking unauthorized leave

It is recommended that the hospital should draw up a procedure to be followed when patients leave hospital contrary to medical advice. The procedure should recognize the different legal category of patients, drawing a distinction between those who have the freedom to leave when they so wish and those who are liable to be detained under the Act or become so liable. The procedure should cover those who should be informed of the patient's departure and the appropriate action which should be taken. If possible, obtain the patient's signature on a form stating that the discharge is taken contrary to medical advice. This will not however protect staff where statutory powers for emergency detention should have been used.

This procedure will become increasingly important in the context of community care since there may be very few homes which are registered to take detained patients. Therefore, if patients leave, the basis on which they are compulsorily returned to the home must be clarified.

Questions and exercises

(1) A patient who is detained under section 3 is found to be missing after he had been given permission to visit the hospital shop. What legal powers exist to force the patient's return to the hospital and what procedures should be followed?

(2) A patient who had been given weekend leave under section 17 to stay with his mother – the nearest relative – refused to return on Monday. The ward sister spoke to the mother who said that the patient was so much better there was no need for him to return to hospital. What action should the ward sister take? What legal powers exist to return the patient to hospital?

(3) A detained patient at X hospital is on section 17 leave at another hospital, Y, which has less secure provision. The ward sister at X is phoned up by a counterpart at Y to request that the patient be taken back. The patient is unwilling to leave Y. What is the law and what procedures should be followed?

(4) A patient was detained on section 5(2) at 8.00PM one Friday evening, but managed to leave the hospital. He remained missing until 7.00PM on Monday night when he was found to be hiding in a friend's house. Could he be legally forced to return to the hospital? What powers exist to force entry into the house?

(5) A severely agitated elderly mentally infirm patient who was not under section wandered off the ward and out of the hospital grounds. She was found in a shopping centre. Could she be legally compelled to return to hospital?

Chapter 12 Entering premises to take a mentally disordered person

Section 135(1) enables a warrant to be obtained to search for and remove patients. The requirements are set out in Figure 12.1. The power under section 135(1) only applies if there is reason to believe that there is a mentally disordered person who is believed to meet the requirements of the section. It does not give a general power of inspection. This is given by section 115 which is set out in Figure 12.2.

Section 135(1)

(1) An approved social worker lays information on oath.

(2) The justice of the peace considers whether there is reasonable cause to suspect that a person believed to be suffering from a mental disorder:
   (a) has been, or is being, ill-treated, neglected or kept otherwise than under proper control, within the jurisdiction of the justice, or
   (b) being unable to care for himself, is living alone in any such place.

(3) If it appears to the justice that there is such reasonable cause he may issue a warrant authorizing any constable*
   (a) to enter, if need be by force, any premises specified in the warrant in which the person is believed to be, and
   (b) to remove him (if thought fit) to a place of safety.

(4) The removal to a place of safety is to be done with a view to making
   (a) an application in respect of him under Part II of the Act (i.e. sections 2, 4 or 3), or
   (b) other arrangements for his treatment or care.

Section 135(3)

(5) A patient who is removed to a place of safety in the execution of a warrant issued under this section may be detained there for a period not exceeding 72 hours.

Section 135(4)

(6) A constable in executing such a warrant **shall*** be accompanied by
    (a) an approved social worker, and
    (b) a registered medical practitioner.

Section 135(5)

(7) The patient need not be named in the warrant.

***Notes** The requirement that the constable should be named in the warrant was removed by the Police and Criminal Evidence Act 1984.
There is a distinction in the requirement that the constable be accompanied between this section 135(1) and section 135(2) (see Figure 11.2).

**Figure 12.1
Searching for and
removing patients –
section 135.**

(1) An approved social worker of a local social services authority may
(2) at all reasonable times
(3) after producing
(4) if asked to do so
(5) some duly authenticated document showing that he is such a social worker
(6) enter and inspect any premises (not being a hospital) in the area of that authority
(7) in which a mentally disordered patient is living
(8) if he has reasonable cause to believe
(9) that the patient is not under proper care.

**Figure 12.2 Power of
entry and inspection of
premises (section 115).**

Section 115 does not give the social worker the power to force entry and therefore if entry is refused a warrant would be required under Section 135 above. Any person refusing entry would of course be committing an offence under section 129.

Section 135(2) gives power on obtaining a warrant to enter premises if need be by force and remove a patient who is liable to be detained under the Act (see Chapter 11).

Questions and exercises

(1) A community psychiatric nurse, who calls regularly on a former detained patient to administer injections, is refused admission. She is concerned about the well-being of the patient. What action should she take? What legal powers if any exist to force entry, inspect the premises and remove the patient?

(2)   A neighbour draws the attention of a community nurse to the fact that the next door neighbour who has had several psychiatric in-patient stays has not been seen for several days and it is feared that she is inside. What should the community nurse do? What is the legal position?

(3)   A patient who is on section 17 leave at home refuses to come to the door when the community psychiatric nurse visits. What is the appropriate action to be taken?

(4)   A patient who is under guardianship has left the specified place of residence and has gone to stay with a friend. What action, if any, can be taken to check his whereabouts and return him to the specified place?

Chapter 13   Police powers of arrest and place of safety

Police powers of arrest

The police have been given specific powers under the Mental Health Act to arrest a person who is believed to be suffering from mental disorder in a place to which the public have access. The requirements are shown in Figure 13.1.

Most districts now have in existence a policy which has been jointly agreed with the health authority, social services and the police.

Section 136(1)

(1) If a constable finds
    (a) in a place to which the public have access
    (b) a person who appears to him
        ● to be suffering from mental disorder **and**
        ● to be in immediate need of care or control

(2) the constable may, if he thinks it necessary to do so
    (a) in the interests of that person or
    (b) for the protection of other persons
    remove that person to a place of safety.

Section 136(2)

(3) A person removed to a place of safety may be detained there for a period not exceeding 72 hours

(4) for the purpose of
    (a) enabling him to be examined by a registered medical practitioner **and**
    (b) enabling him to be interviewed by an approved social worker **and**
    (c) making any necessary arrangements for his treatment or care.

Note Many of these provisions are linked by '**and**' rather than '**or**'. This means that they must **all** be satisfied.

Figure 13.1 Police powers of arrest.

Place of safety

There is considerable local variation in what is agreed to be the usual place of safety: sometimes the policy envisages that the patient will normally be brought to the hospital, sometimes the place of safety is the police station. Figure 13.2 sets out the statutory provisions on the place of safety.

Figure 13.2 Place of safety – section 135(6).

- Residential accommodation provided by a local social services authority under Part III of the National Assistance Act 1948.
- Residential accommodation provided by a local social services authority under paragraph 2 of Schedule 8 of the National Health Service Act 1977.
- A hospital as defined by section 145(1) of the Act.
- A police station.
- A mental nursing home or residential home for mentally disordered persons.
- Any other suitable place the occupier of which is willing temporarily to receive the patient.

There are no statutory forms to be completed in respect of the use of section 136. Many hospitals have therefore designed their own. A specimen is shown in Appendix II (Example G). The advantage of using such a form is that it records the basis of the patient's detention in the hospital, the name of the constable who brought the patient to the hospital and the time of the patient's arrival.

Problems with section 136

Section 136 has not been without difficulties in its implementation and the following are some of the queries which have arisen on its use.

Q1. *What if the police sergeant decides that it is not necessary for the patient to be seen by an approved social worker or by a registered doctor?*

A1. The Act does not appear to give him this discretion if it is necessary to detain the patient at the place of safety. Once arrested the patient's detention is for the purpose of an examination being carried out by the approved social worker and the doctor.

Q2. *If a police station is used as the place of safety can the patient be transferred elsewhere under the powers given by section 136?*

A2. There is no decided case upon this and the Act interpreted strictly would not appear to give this power. The 72 hour period commences with the arrival at the place of safety and there does not seem to be the opportunity for consecutive places of safety for the same patient to be organized all under section 136. If following the assessment and examination it is decided that the patient should be detained then there would have to be an application under Part II of the Act. This shows how important it is to have an agreed place of safety in the local policy which covers every eventuality.

Q3. *What issues arise if, as is not unknown, a police officer arrests a person in a public place and brings him to the police station when the duty officer decides that this constitutes a section 136 arrest and arranges for the police to take the patient to the hospital?*

A3. Should the nurse be confronted with this situation, the following points should be noted.
- If the patient refuses to stay, and has not been admitted as an in-patient, there is no power to use section 5(2) (application for admission) or section 5(4) (Nurse's Holding Power).
- If the patient leaves the hospital, the patient cannot be returned to the hospital under section 138 which would be the provision which applied to a person lawfully detained under section 136.

Q4. *If a patient absconds from the place of safety what are the powers of retaking?*

A4. Section 137 deems a person who is being conveyed to a place of safety or is at the place of safety to be in legal custody. Section 138 gives the power for the patient to be retaken if he absconds from the place of safety or from legal custody. However the person cannot be retaken after the expiration of 72 hours beginning with the time when he escapes or the period during which he is liable to be so detained, whichever expires first (section 138(3)).

Q5. *What if the registered medical practitioner refuses to attend the place of safety?*

A5. If this should occur the police have no option other than to arrange for a doctor to come since this is a requirement under the Act. A local policy will set out how the doctor is to be obtained and also will usually set up arrangements for a rota system. Increasingly purchasing authorities are including, in their NHS agreements with providers, duties under the Mental

Health Act and setting targets e.g. the time within which the provider should arrange for a registered doctor to arrive at the place of safety. Seventy two hours is the maximum time that a person can be kept under section 136, and usually the time should be much less since, as soon as the assessment and the examination have been completed and the arrangements made for his treatment or care, the section should cease.

Q6. *If the patient needs medication can this be given under section 136?*

A6. The answer to this is that section 136 patients are excluded from the provisions of Part IV of the Act relating to consent to treatment. This means that there is no statutory power to compel treatment to be taken. Only in a very dire emergency, when it could be argued that the best interests of the patient require that treatment be given, could common law powers be used (see Chapter 8).

Q7. *What information should be given to a person detained under section 136?*

A7. If a police station is used as the place of safety there is no statutory duty under section 132 for information to be given (see Chapter 6). However there is a duty under the Police and Criminal Evidence Act 1984 to allow the person to have another person of his choice informed of his arrest and whereabouts following an arrest under 136 and, if he is in a police station, he has a right to legal advice.

Monitoring of section 136

Because of the problems in the past with this section there should be careful monitoring of its use and the joint policy should be reviewed in the light of the results of the monitoring. The monitoring should take account of the features listed in Figure 13.3.

(1) Frequency of use.
(2) Outcomes of assessment and examination.
(3) Time of notification to approved social worker and doctor.
(4) Time of arrival of approved social worker and doctor.
(5) Length of detention.
(6) Suitability of the chosen places of safety.
(7) Any other problems which have arisen in its use.

Figure 13.3 Features to be considered in monitoring section 136.

Questions and exercises

(1) A police constable brings a patient to hospital purportedly under section 136 after he had been arrested during a very raucous party. Neighbours had summoned the police. Does the ward sister have to accept the admission? The patient is unwilling to stay.

(2) What do you consider should be a reasonable target within which the approved social worker and the doctor should assess and examine the patient at the place of safety following arrest under section 136?

(3) Discuss whether or not a place of safety should normally be a hospital.

(4) A patient has been brought to hospital by the police under section 136. The doctor recommends that treatment should be given immediately but the patient refuses to consent. What legal powers exist, if any, to compel the patient to have treatment?

(5) A patient is brought to the hospital as a place of safety under section 136 and he leaves the hospital. What rights exist to return the patient to hospital and who would be permitted to bring him back? (See Chapter 11.)

Chapter 14   Transfer of patients

Detained patients

The Act makes provision for detained patients to be transferred from one hospital to another or into the guardianship of a local social services authority, or from guardianship to another local social services authority or to hospital. Section 19 sets out the provisions; details are given in Figures 14.1, 14.2, 14.3, and 14.4.

Further detailed regulations are set out in the Mental Health (Hospital, Guardianship and Consent to Treatment) Regulations 1983 (SI 1983 No. 893), paragraphs 7 to 9. The functions of the managers may be performed by an officer authorized by them in that regard (Regulations, paragraph 7(5)). Paragraph 9 of these Regulations is headed 'Conveyance to hospital or transfer' and covers the time limits and people involved. Figure 14.5 summarizes the rules on time limits and people involved in transference of patients.

The requirements are summarized diagrammatically in Figures 14.6 and 14.7.

(1) Provisions cover patients detained by virtue of an application and therefore do not cover patients detained under sections 5(2) and 5(4) (emergency holding powers), 135 and 136 (police powers of arrest), or 35, 36 and 38 (criminal provisions). Patients under section 37 can be transferred (Sched. 1, Part 1, para 2 and 5) and patients under section 37/41 restriction can be transferred with the consent of the Secretary of State (Sched. 1, Part 2, para 2 and 5).

(2) Following the transfer, the original date of detention is treated as if the patient was originally admitted to the new hospital at that time.

(3) Any patient detained under Part II of the Act can be transferred to other hospitals under the same managers. No form is required (section 19(3)).

(4) Regulation 7 requires that an 'authority to transfer' as set out in Part I of Form 24 is given by the managers of the hospital in which the patient is liable to be detained.

(5) Those managers must be satisfied that arrangements have been made for the admission of the patient to the hospital to which he is being transferred within a period of 28 days beginning with the date of the authority for transfer.

(6) On the transfer the managers must record his admission as set out in Part II of Form 24.

Figure 14.1 Transfers of patients detained by virtue of an application.

(1) These provisions do not cover patients on section 5(2), 5(4), 135 and 136.

(2) Following the transfer the patient is treated as though he were placed under guardianship on the date of the original detention.

(3) The patient may be transferred into the guardianship of the local social services authority or of any person approved by that authority.

(4) The managers of the hospital in which the patient is detained complete Part I of Form 25.

(5) The transfer must be agreed by the local social services authority which will be responsible as set out in Part II of Form 25.

(6) The local social services authority must specify the date on which the transfer shall take place.

(7) Where a person other than the social services authority is to be the guardian that person must agree and record that agreement on Part III of Form 25.

Figure 14.2 Transfers into guardianship.

(1) An authority for transfer must be given by the guardian as set out in Part I of Form 26.

(2) The transfer must be agreed by the local social services authority as set out in Part II of Form 26.

(3) The local social services authority must specify the date on which the transfer shall take place.

(4) The agreement of the proposed guardian (where this is not the local social services authority) must be obtained and set out as in Part III of Form 26.

Figure 14.3 Transfer from guardianship to guardianship.

Figure 14.4 Transfer from guardianship to hospital.

(1) Authority can be given by the local social services authority in Form 27 in the following circumstances.

   (a) An application for treatment has been made by an approved social worker in the form set out in Form 9.
   (b) The social worker must have consulted the nearest relative (section 11(4)) and carried out the duties under section 13.
   (c) The application must be founded on two medical recommendations in accordance with section 12 on either Form 28 or 29.
   (d) The application must be accepted by the managers of the hospital to which it is addressed, and the local social services authority must be satisfied that arrangements have been made for the admission of the patient within the period of 14 days beginning with the date of the authority for transfer.
   (e) The responsible local social services authority must take such steps as are practicable to inform the person (if any) appearing to be the patient's nearest relative of the proposed transfer.

(2) On the transfer of the patient a record of admission shall be made by the managers of the hospital to which he is being transferred in the form set out in Form 14 and shall be attached to the application.

Figure 14.5 Time limits for transfer of patients.

(1) Transfer between hospitals must take place within the period of 28 days beginning with the authority for transfer (Regulation 9(1)(a) of SI 1983 No. 893).

(2) Transfer from guardianship to hospital must take place within the period of 14 days beginning with the date on which the patient was last examined by a medical practitioner for the purposes of transfer (Regulation 9(1)(b) of SI 1983 No. 893).

Informal patients

There are no statutory provisions governing the voluntary transfer of informal patients from hospital to hospital. However, with the introduction of the internal market, it is important to distinguish between transfers **within** the direction of the Trust or Directly Managed Unit of the hospital where the patient is detained and transfers **outside**. Where the transfer is outside, and the patient's case will count as an extra-contractual referral, then the purchaser's consent to the transfer **must** be obtained

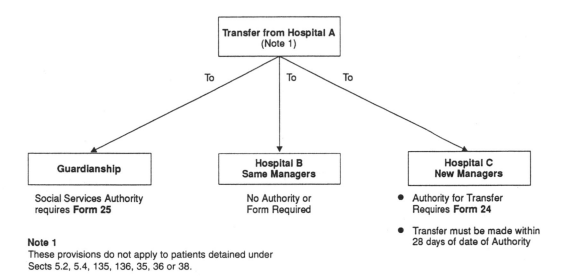

Figure 14.6   Transfer of patients from hospital.

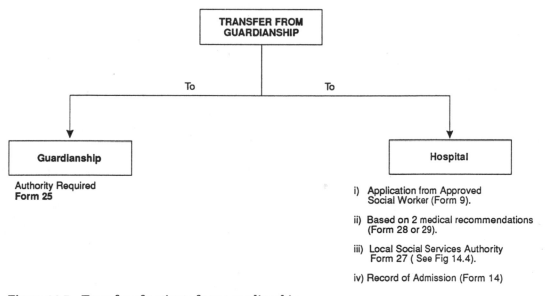

Figure 14.7   Transfer of patients from guardianship.

before arrangements are finalized. The purchaser may be the health authority or, in the case of a patient in a general practice which is fund-holding, the fund-holders.

Informal patients can be transferred between hospitals with their consent and, if necessary, with the agreement of the purchasers. If the patient is incapable of giving valid consent,

consent can be given by the relative acting in the patient's best interests. Transfers from NHS to non-NHS accommodation may lead to fees being charged to the patient, and the Department of Health has laid down guidance on such transfers.

Questions and exercises

(1) You are the primary nurse for a patient who is due to be transferred to a nursing home for the mentally disordered registered to take detained patients. The section is to continue. What procedures must be followed to ensure that the legal requirements are met? What would be the situation if the nursing home was not registered to take detained patients?

(2) You are on an admission ward when a detained patient transferred from another hospital is admitted. There appears to be no statutory documents with him. What should be there and what action would you take? What difference would it make if the patient was under a restriction order?

Chapter 15 Guardianship

There were hopes that, following the changes to the guardianship law, more use would be made of this section by social services authorities in order to provide supervised care for patients outside the institutions. In general these hopes have not been fulfilled though some authorities have made greater use of it than others.

What are the statutory provisions?

Figure 15.1 sets out the grounds for a guardianship application. Like an application under section 3 (admission for treatment) it must be shown that one of the specific forms of mental disorder exists and the two medical recommendations must have one in common irrespective of whether other forms of mental disorder also exist.

Figure 15.1 Medical conditions for guardianship – section 7.

(1) Patient is suffering from mental disorder, being mental illness, severe mental impairment, psychopathic disorder or mental impairment and his mental disorder is of a nature or degree which warrants his reception into guardianship under this section; and

(2) it is necessary in the interests of the welfare of the patient or for the protection of other persons that the patient should be so received.

A person must be 16 or over to be received into guardianship. The application must state the age of the person, or if the exact age is not known that the patient is believed to be over 16 years.

Guardianship can also be ordered by the court under section 37.

Who can make an application?

The nearest relative or an approved social worker can be an applicant (section 11(1)).

Duration

Like admission for treatment the guardianship order can last initially for up to 6 months, can be renewed for a further 6 months and then can be renewed for twelve months at a time.

Procedure

The application is to be forwarded to the local social services authority within a period of 14 days beginning with the date on which the patient was last examined by a registered medical practitioner before giving a medical recommendation for the purposes of guardianship (section 8(2)).

Powers of a guardian

Under the previous law the guardian had all the powers of a father over a child of 14. Under the 1983 Act the powers are more specific and are set out in Figure 15.2.

---

(1) The power to require the patient to reside at a place specified by the authority or person named as guardian.

(2) The power to require the patient to attend at places and times so specified for the purpose of medical treatment, occupation, education or training.

(3) The power to require that access to the patient be given, at any place where the patient is residing, to any registered medical practitioner, approved social worker or other person so specified.

Figure 15.2 Powers of a guardian – section 8(1).

These powers are limited and, apart from the right to return the patient to the specified place under section 18(3), unenforceable. The provisions of section 18(3) are set out in Figure 15.3.

Who is the guardian?

The person named as the guardian may be the local social services authority or any other person including the applicant. Where the guardian is not the local social services authority then that nomination must be accepted on behalf of that person by the local social services authority for the area in which he resides. In addition the named person must complete a statement in writing that he is willing to act as a guardian (section 7(5)).

Section 18(3)
> Where a patient who is for the time being subject to guardianship under this Part of this Act
>
> - absents himself without the leave of the guardian
> - from the place at which he is required by the guardian to reside,
>
> he may be taken into custody and returned to that place
>
> - by any constable, or
> - by any person authorized in writing by the guardian or a local social services authority.

Section 18(4)
> If however the patient has been away from the specified place for 28 days or more without leave, then he cannot be retaken and ceases to be subject to guardianship.

Figure 15.3 Return of patient under guardianship – section 18(3).

Duties of a guardian

These are set out in the Mental Health (Hospital, Guardianship and Consent to Treatment) Regulations 1983 (SI 1983 No. 893) and shown in Figure 15(4).

The local social services authority as guardian

An application for guardianship may nominate the local social services authority as the guardian. Where this authority is the guardian it has similar responsibilities to the private guardian and has the same powers set out in section 8 (see Figure 15.2). In addition where a person acting as a private guardian becomes incapacitated or dies or makes known a request not to remain as guardian, the local social services authority would have a duty to take over responsibilities of guardianship until another guardian is appointed.

Transfer of patients from and into guardianship

A patient who is liable to be detained in a hospital can be transferred into guardianship of a local social services authority or of any person approved by such an authority (section 19(1)(a)).

A patient who is subject to guardianship may be transferred

It shall be the duty of a private guardian:

(1) to appoint a registered medical practitioner to act as the nominated medical attendant of the patient;

(2) to notify the responsible local social services authority of the name and address of the nominated medical attendant;

(3) in exercising the powers and duties conferred or imposed upon him by the Act and these Regulations, to comply with such directions as that authority may give;

(4) to furnish that authority with all such reports or other information with regard to the patient as the authority may from time to time require;

(5) to notify the authority:
  (a) on the reception of the patient into guardianship, of his address and the address of the patient;
  (b) except in a case to which paragraph (6) applies, of any permanent change of either address, before or not later than 7 days after the change takes place;

(6) where on any permanent change of his address, the new address is in the area of a different local social services authority, to notify that authority:
  (a) of his address and that of the patient,
  (b) of the particulars mentioned in (2),
  and to send a copy of the notification to the authority which was formerly responsible; and

(7) in the event of the death of the patient, or the termination of the guardianship by discharge, transfer or otherwise, to notify the responsible local social services authority as soon as reasonably practicable.

Figure 15.4 Duties of guardian – paragraph 12, SI 1983 No. 893.

into the guardianship of another social services authority or person, or be transferred to a hospital (section 19(1)(b)).

Following the transfer, the patient is deemed to have been in the new situation from the time the original application was accepted (for further details see Chapter 14). The Mental Health (Hospital, Guardianship and Consent to Treatment) Regulations 1983, SI 1983 No. 893 provide the detailed rules.

Questions and exercises

(1) Identify the powers of the guardian. Do you think that they should be expanded or reduced?

(2)   Why do you think that there has been such erratic use of the guardianship provisions of the Act across the country?

(3)   The approved social worker and the responsible medical officer are of the opinion that a patient currently subject to section 3 could be transferred into guardianship. What procedures must be followed?

(1)   You are a community psychiatric nurse and are aware that a patient who is subject to guardianship is not taking his medication. What action could you take?

(5)   What would you consider to be the advantages and disadvantages of giving the guardian the right to agree to the patient being giving compulsory treatment in the community?

Chapter 16 The role of the approved social worker and the social worker

The approved social worker was a new concept under the 1983 Act. Specific statutory duties were given to those social workers who had completed an approved course of training.

As the main source of applications for admission under the Act (since applications by the nearest relative are few), the approved social worker has a major role to perform in the care of the mentally disordered. However there are other statutory duties to be performed which can be undertaken by a social worker who is not necessarily approved and this chapter covers these duties as well.

Powers and duties of the approved social worker

Figure 16.1 sets out the powers of the approved social worker.

Section 115	Power to enter and inspect any non-hospital premises.
Section 135(1)	Power to apply for warrant to enter premises and remove patient.
Section 135(2)	Power to apply for warrant to enter premises and remove patient who is liable to be taken into custody.
Section 18	Power to take into custody and return patient absent without leave.
Section 138	Power to retake patients escaping from custody.
Section 11(1)	Power to apply for the admission of patient or admission into guardianship.
Section 13(3)	Power to apply for the admission into guardianship of patient outside the area of the local social service authority by which the social worker has been appointed.
Section 29(2)	Power to initiate appointment by court of acting nearest relative by applying for a court order directing that the function of the nearest relative be exercisable by the local social services authority or by any other specified person.

Figure 16.1 Powers of the approved social worker.

The duties of the approved social worker, as stipulated in various sections of the Act, are set out in Figure 16.2.

Section 11(3)	The approved social worker must take such steps as are practicable to **inform** the nearest relative of the admission of the patient for assessment (sections 2 and 4) and of the nearest relative's right of discharge. This information must be given before or within a **reasonable** time after an application has been made.
Section 11(4)	The approved social worker **must consult** with the person appearing to be the nearest relative of the patient before an application for admission for treatment (section 3) or an application for guardianship (section 7) is made.

Note
- This does not apply if it appears to the approved social worker that in the circumstances such consultation is not reasonably practicable or would involve unreasonable delay.
- If the nearest relative objects to the application it cannot be made.

Section 13(4)	An approved social worker must

- if directed by the local social services authority
- if required by the nearest relative,

as soon as practicable take the patient's case into consideration with a view to making an application for his admission to hospital.

Note
The approved social worker shall inform the nearest relative of his reasons in writing if he decides not to make an application.

Section 13(1)	An approved social worker should apply for an admission to hospital or guardianship for a patient within the area of his appointment where he is satisfied

- that such an application ought to be made, and
- that it is necessary or proper for the application to be made by him having regard to the wishes expressed by the relatives of the patient or any other relevant circumstances.

Section 13(2)   An approved social worker shall
- interview the patient in a suitable manner and
- satisfy himself that detention in a hospital is in all the circumstances of the case the most appropriate way of providing the care and medical treatment the patient needs

before making an application for admission to hospital.

Figure 16.2 Duties of the approved social worker.

Duties of any social worker

Figure 16.3 sets out those statutory duties which can be performed by any social worker within the appropriate area.

Section 14   To provide a report on social circumstances where a patient is admitted to hospital on an application **by the nearest relative** (other than an emergency application under section 4).

- The managers must give notice of the fact as soon as practicable to the local social services authority for the area in which the patient resided immediately before admission.
- The authority must arrange as soon as practicable for a social worker of their department to interview the patient and provide the managers with a report on his social circumstances.

Section 117   Duty of district health authority and of the local social services authority to provide after-care services (see Chapter 17).

Figure 16.3 Duties of any social worker.

Medical recommendations

Unless approved social workers are satisfied that the medical recommendations are sufficient to justify the compulsory admission of any patient as an in-patient, they should not apply for the admission of the patient. The approved social worker therefore provides the first check on the adequacy of the recommendations for admission discussed in Chapter 3. If the nurse is also concerned about any particular recommendation, she could discuss it with the approved social worker.

The nurse and the social worker

It is essential that social workers should be involved in the multi-disciplinary care of the patient. This should happen not only prior to the admission when the approved social worker, rather than the nearest relative, is likely to be the applicant, but also during the hospital stay and in preparing for discharge. This should apply not only to those patients who come under the provisions of section 117 (see Chapter 17) but to all patients including the informal patient. Nurses are in the best position to ensure that there is full involvement of the social services personnel who will be dependent upon ward staff to notify them of relevant ward meetings etc. Unfortunately the structure and organization of mental health social services is not always the most appropriate for linking in with hospital care, and in such areas more conscious effort is required from ward staff to ensure that the social services personnel are notified of appropriate meetings and their help sought when required by a patient.

In some districts the community mental health services provided by social services is linked in very closely with health authority/NHS trust provision. Social services might for example share office accommodation with community psychiatric nursing staff within a community mental health home. Sometimes, too, general practitioners provide services to these homes, thus facilitating communication across the artificial barriers of the structure of health service care, Family Health Services Authority services and social services. Eventually the close cooperation of these groups might lead the way to new organizational statutory structures based on primary care teams.

At present it is essential that the nurse has a good understanding of the role and responsibilities of both the approved social worker and the social worker. Rehabilitation may be facilitated if the social worker is closely involved in the treatment plan of the patient and is able to discuss the social and financial issues relating to discharge at an early stage. In addition the approved social worker might be called upon as the second professional to be consulted by the second opinion appointed doctor before he recommends whether treatment should be given without the patient's consent. Unless social workers have been professionally concerned with the care of the patient, they could not undertake this consultative role. If they are so involved, they can be invaluable members of the team.

Questions and exercises

(1)   What part do you consider the approved social worker should play in the multi-disciplinary team?

(2)   A patient tells you that he wishes for personal reasons to have another approved social worker. Are there any legal restrictions on this being changed?

(3)   An approved social worker fails to consult the nearest relative before applying for section 3 admission. What defences does he have?

Chapter 17 Community care

The provision of community care has long been a partnership of the health authorities, local social services authorities, voluntary groups, private organizations and the family and carers of the patient, with probably the bulk of the responsibility and financing falling upon the family. Statutory duties exist for both health and local authorities to provide community care: the National Health Service and Community Care Act 1990 has given added responsibilities to local social services authorities to establish assessment of needs and provision of services. The possibility of any individual enforcing these statutory duties under the 1990 Act has not yet come to court. The duties apply to all mentally disordered clients as well as to those with other disabilities. The 'care programme approach' was implemented on 1 April 1993. There is considerable disquiet over the resourcing and the full financial implications, and some authorities have claimed they are in danger of not meeting their statutory responsibilities (Surrey County Council in January 1995 requested registered homes to provide a free place until resources become available).

Detained patients

There is a statutory duty on health authorities and local social service authorities to plan the after-care of certain detained patients. Section 117 applies to those patients shown in Figure 17.1.

The duty consists in the health and local authorities agreeing with voluntary agencies to provide after-care services for any person under this section. The duty lasts until both the authorities are satisfied that the person concerned is no longer in need

Figure 17.1 Patients covered by statutory after-care provisions.

- Patients detained under section 3.
- Patients admitted under section 37.
- Patients transferred under section 47 or 48.

of such services. In 1993 a patient brought a successful action against a local health authority for failure to provide section 117 services (*R* v. *Ealing District Health Authority, ex parte Fox* (1993)) (see Glossary).

It is highly desirable that the after-care planning should begin as soon as possible, perhaps even before the patient's admission. The Code of Practice gives guidance on the procedures to be followed and the staff who should be involved in the discussions (see Chapter 27 of the Code of Practice). It is also essential that the carers and relatives should be involved at an early stage in the after-care planning. Section 17 leave (see Chapter 10) should also be planned in the context of an overall treatment plan which includes after-care.

A typical form for implementing section 117 is given in outline in Appendix II, Example H. The full form is 13 pages in length and includes:

Appendix 1 Notification of entitlement to After-care
Appendix 2 Individual Information and Discharge Plan
Appendix 3 Individual Discharge Plan – Checklist
Appendix 4 Refusal of After-care
Appendix 5 Reports by Key Worker following 6 months discharge from hospital
Appendix 6 Notification of discharge from Section 117
Appendix 7 Case Conference (Notification to Medical Secretary)
Appendix 8 Case Conference (Notification to Participants)

What if the detained patient refuses after-care?

There is no provision in the Act for after-care to be given compulsorily, so, even though it is highly desirable for a patient to receive treatment or supervision after discharge, there is no power to force this upon the patient. Does the duty therefore terminate as a result of the patient's refusal?

The section envisages that the duty will end when both the District Health Authority and the local social services authority are satisfied that the person concerned is no longer in need of such services. This is not the case if the patient is refusing help. The correct approach in such cases is probably for the patient to continue to be monitored and such contact kept. If he eventually decides to accept after-care then assistance can be provided.

Section 117 and the care programme approach

In many areas the planning and procedures for section 117 have become subsumed in the implementation of the care programme approach which arises from duties placed on local social services authorities under the National Health Service and Community Care Act 1990. The care programme approach covers a much wider group of the mentally disordered than section 117 and also covers other disabilities.

However the statutory duty under section 117 exists in parallel with the care programme approach and must still be fulfilled.

The nurse and the after-care planning

The nurse is an essential member of the multi-disciplinary team which prepares for the patient's after-care. Where possible it is advisable for the community psychiatric nurse who is likely to be involved in the patient's care in the community also to take part in the discussions since this should assist in the continuity of care.

It should be possible to identify gaps in the provision of community services which result in the patient staying in hospital longer than his clinical condition requires. This information is also obtained from an analysis of the reasons given in the medical recommendations for admission to hospital.

Feeding such information into the strategic planning for the care programme approach should enable the purchasers of health services and the local social services authorities to define where the gaps exist and make contracts for provision in the future.

Background to the Mental Health (Patients in the Community) Act 1995

The Royal College of Psychiatrists' Report

The absence of a power to treat patients compulsorily has led to a suggestion that the Act should be amended to permit some form of community order or community supervision. The suggestion has arisen from the concern about the numbers of chronic patients who on discharge into the community fail to keep up with the treatment regimes and eventually have to be returned to hospital for compulsory treatment, thus creating what has been termed the 'revolving door'.

A report of the Royal College of Psychiatrists (January 1993) proposed a new community supervision order. This would enable patients to be cared for in their homes. It was based on six principles as shown in Figure 17.2.

(1) It is undesirable to give compulsory treatment in the community without consent.

(2) Compulsory supervision in the community is in the interests of a limited and defined group of patients.

(3) Compulsory arrangements in the community must have safeguards and must not be used as an alternative to circumventing community care.

(4) Arrangements should not be open ended.

(5) The grounds for compulsory arrangements should be clear.

(6) There should be opportunities to apply for a discharge from such an order.

Figure 17.2 Principles – new Community Supervision Order.

These principles overcame many of the objections which were voiced over earlier proposals which seemed to suggest that the community psychiatric nurse might have been involved in the giving of compulsory treatment in the community. Nor do the proposals place additional burdens upon the guardian.

The Select Committee Report

The House of Commons Select Committee reported in June 1993 on community supervision orders (*Health Committee Session 1992–93, Fifth Report*). Its conclusions were that it could not support the College's proposals. Instead it suggested making fully effective the present statutory and non-statutory provisions for the care of people with a mental illness. It did not recommend any changes in the guardianship provisions until more was known about the reasons for their restricted use. It recommended that the suggestion for the use of crisis cards should be examined. It supported the Mental Health Act Commission's recommendation for a review of the Act.

Department of Health Internal Inquiry

The Department of Health set up an internal inquiry into the legal powers on the care of the mentally ill in the community which reported in August 1993. This inquiry recommended that active consideration should be given to extending the powers of guardianship, to removing the six month limit on section 17 and to the introduction of a supervised discharge power over non-restricted patients who present a risk following discharge. These recommendations were included in the Mental Health (Patients in the Community) Act 1995 (see below).

Interim progress   In August 1993, the Secretary of State for Health announced a package of measures to reinforce the care in the community for mentally ill persons. These did not apply to Wales. They included the following.

- Firstly, a new power of supervised discharge for mentally ill people who need special support. Legislation was required for this and a Bill was introduced in the 1995 Session of Parliament.

- Secondly, a supervision register for those in a special category of risk. This came into force in April 1994 on the basis of guidance issued in December 1993:

  '... from April 1994 it will be for the health authorities to ensure through their contracts that providers draw up and maintain proper registers. This will identify those potentially at risk to themselves or others and help ensure that the Care Programme Approach is backed by rigorous monitoring.' (Secretary of State, December 1993).

Guidelines for discharge were issued by the Department of Health in January 1994. They give guidance on:

- the criteria to take into account in deciding on discharge;
- the implementation of the care programme approach and section 117 duties;
- dealing with patients who present special risks; and
- action to be taken if things go wrong.

The report following the murder by Christopher Clunis, a patient with a chronic history of mental illness, highlighted some of the major deficiencies in providing after-care and continuity of care.

In 1994 the Audit Commission *Finding a Place – A Review of Mental Health Service for Adults* (HMSO 1994), concluded that a clear strategy set out in jointly agreed plans was required to meet the needs of the mentally ill adults in the community. It put forward eleven recommendations for purchasers and providers to ensure the deficiencies which existed are remedied and it set down action plans for

- central government,
- district purchasers,

- purchasers and providers,
- provider managers,
- FHSAs,
- GPs and primary care teams,
- social services and
- housing agencies.

Nurses should obtain sight of this Audit report and ensure that they play their full part in the implementation of its recommendations. From 1 April 1996 FHSAs and HAs are replaced by new health authorities (Health Services Act 1995).

Mental Health (Patients in the Community) Act 1995

This bill went through Parliament in 1995 to provide a system of supervision of the care in the community of certain patients who have been detained in hospital under the mental health legislation. In England and Wales after-care supervision is to be provided; in Scotland community care orders are to be set up. The 1995 Act also extended the period under which leave of absence can be granted by removing the 1983 Act six month limit. It also extended the period under which certain patients who are absent without leave can be taken into custody. It came into force on 1 April 1996.

Extracts from the Act are shown in Appendix I(B).

Questions and exercises

(1) How soon do you think planning for after-care should begin?

(2) Consider some of the difficulties in arranging potential after-care and how they could be resolved?

(3) There is a danger that inadequate resources are used as a scapegoat for other deficiencies in after-care planning. What might these deficiencies be?

(4) An approved social worker complains that she only knows that a patient is due to be discharged when she finds that he is actually in the community. How do you think the after-care planning could be improved in such cases?

(5) Discuss the advantages and disadvantages of the Community Supervision Order as suggested by the Royal College of Psychiatrists.

(6) Extracts from the Mental Health (Patients in the Community) Act 1995 are given in Appendix I(B). Consider these and discuss how they can be implemented.

Chapter 18 Rectification of documents

In Chapter 3, which deals with the definition of mental disorder and medical recommendation, we considered briefly the possibility of rectifying documents and the limitations on rectifying the documents relating to the medical recommendations. This chapter will deal with document scrutiny and rectification generally. It might be thought that minor errors on forms can be changed at any time and are of little significance, but these documents are the legal basis for the detention of the patient and the managers have a direct responsibility to ensure that they are scrutinized as correct and that appropriate steps are taken for them to be rectified if necessary. Any person who alters a document other than as permitted by law would be committing an offence under section 126 (see Chapter 21) as would anyone who permitted the use of such documents.

Rectification under the Act

Permitted rectifications

Figure 18.1 sets out the provisions of section 15(1) which permits rectification in certain circumstances.

An application or recommendation can only be amended:

- if the application, or any medical recommendation given for the purposes of the application, is found to be in any respect incorrect or defective,

- within the period of 14 days beginning with the day on which a patient has been admitted to hospital in pursuance of an application for admission for assessment or for treatment,

- with the consent of the managers of the hospital, and

- by the person by whom it is signed.

Note Upon such amendment being made the application or recommendation shall be deemed to have had the effect as if it had been originally made as so amended.

Figure 18.1 Rectification – provisions of section 15(1).

Forbidden rectification

Rectification **cannot** take place in the circumstances shown in Figure 18.2.

(1) If there is no signature.

(2) If the medical recommendations do not include a specific form of mental disorder which is mentioned in common.

(3) If the statutory time limits are exceeded.

(4) If a signatory is not empowered to be such under the Act, e.g. the doctor is excluded under section 12, the social worker is not approved, the applicant purports to be the nearest relative but the signatory is not in fact the nearest relative as defined in section 26.

(5) If 14 days have elapsed since the patient was admitted.

(6) If the managers refuse their consent to the rectification.

Figure 18.2 Situations where rectification cannot take place.

A period of only 14 days after admission is permitted for rectification to take place. After that time if the documents are inaccurate the patient would be illegally detained and an application for admission would have to begin afresh.

The managers could refuse to give consent for the documents to be rectified. Normally this is unlikely but if there seems to be a casualness on the part of those who complete forms who think that they will be checked and therefore great care need not be taken in completing them, the managers could take a stand and refuse to allow the documents to be rectified. In this case a new application would have to be started.

If the application relates to section 4 (emergency admission) it cannot be rectified under section 15 after it has expired unless it has been converted into an application for assessment under section 4(4).

Typical errors

Figure 18.3 sets out the kind of errors which could be amended under section 15.

(1) Leaving blank any of the spaces on the form.

(2) Failure to delete one or more alternatives.

(3) Patient's forename and surname not agreeing in different places on documents.

Figure 18.3 Rectification – kinds of error which can be amended.

The procedure for rectification would be for the managers to ensure that a scrutiny takes place as soon as the statutory documents have been received. Any incorrect documents must be returned to the signatory for amendment as soon as possible so that they can be returned within 14 days from the date of admission. The documents would then be scrutinized again and, if correct, formally received. The consent of the manager to this rectification should be given in writing.

Failure to rectify within the 14 day time limit

What is the legal situation if errors have occurred which could have been rectified within 14 days, but they are not spotted in time? For example, a doctor has failed to give the full name and address. The effect of the error is to render the admission illegal. Fresh recommendations and application would be needed to detain the patient. The patient would become informal in the meantime.

Check-lists for certain forms of application

Check-lists for the different applications are given in Figures 18.4 to 18.8.

(1) Is there a doctor's holding order on Form 12?

(2) Is the order signed?

(3) Has the diary date been raised? (72 hours from the time of signature)

(4) Has the patient been informed of his/her rights?

(5) Has the nearest relative been informed?

(6) Has the social work department been informed?

(7) Have the managers received the report on Form 14?

(8) For later monitoring:
- At what time was the assessment carried out by the doctor and the approved social worker?
- Was an application completed in respect of section 2 or section 3?
- Did the patient become informal after the assessment had taken place?
- How long did the section continue? (Note: The section should not be allowed to continue for the full 72 hours: there should be a positive decision taken to admit under section or discontinue the order.)

Figure 18.4   Check-list – section 5(2).

(1)   Is there a nurse's holding order on Form 13?

(2)   Is the form signed by a registered nurse of the prescribed class?

(3)   Is there a Form 16 certifying lapse of the order?

(4)   Is Form 16 signed by the prescribed nurse?

(5)   For later monitoring:

- How long was the patient detained under section 5(4)?
- How frequently was the doctor's holding power used under section 5(2)?
- Were there any occasions when the doctor failed to arrive and the order lapsed through time? What were the reasons?
- How long on average did the doctor take to come? Is this acceptable?

Figure 18.5   Check-list – section 5(4).

(1)   Is there an application by the approved social worker on Form 6 or by the nearest relative on Form 5?

(2)   If the application has been made by the nearest relative have social services been informed?

(3)   Is the application signed?

(4)   Has the applicant seen the patient within the 24 hours ending with the time of the application?

(5)   Is there one medical recommendation on Form 7?

(6)   Is the medical recommendation signed by a doctor who has previous acquaintance with the patient?

(7)   If not, has this been explained on Form 6?

(8)   Do the details on the medical recommendation correspond with the application form?

(9)   Is the date of admission within the period of 24 hours beginning with the time of examination by the recommending doctor or the time of the application whichever is earlier?

(10) Has the patient been informed of his rights both by word of mouth and in writing? Is a record kept of the patient's level of understanding?

(11) Has the nearest relative been given the statutory information in writing?

(12) If not, has the patient requested in writing that the nearest relative should not be informed?

(13) Has the diary date been raised?

(14) Has the medical recommendation been scrutinized by another consultant?

(15) For future monitoring:

- How long did the section last?
- What was the outcome?
- How frequently was a doctor who did not know the patient making the recommendation?
- How often was the nearest relative rather than the approved social worker the applicant?
- What was the outcome?

(16) Have forms 14 and 15 been completed correctly?

Figure 18.6 Checklist – section 4 (emergency application for admission for assessment).

(1) Is there an application by an approved social worker on Form 2 or is there an application by the nearest relative on Form 1?

(2) Have the social services been informed for the home circumstances report?

(3) Is the application signed?

(4) Is the date on which the applicant last saw the patient within 14 days of the application?

(5) Is there a joint medical recommendation on Form 3, **or** are there two medical recommendations each on a separate Form 4?

(6) Is one of the medical recommendations signed by a doctor who was previously acquainted with the patient? If not does the form contain an explanation?

(7) Is one of the medical recommendations signed by a doctor approved for the purpose of section 12?

(8) Where the doctors have examined the patient separately did more than five days elapse between the days on which the separate examinations took place?

(9) Are the dates of the signature of both medical recommendations on or before the date of the application?

(10) If both doctors work at the same hospital is the responsible medical officer (RMO) aware of section 12(4) of the Act? (part-time doctor at the same hospital)

(11) Do the details on the medical recommendations correspond with the application form?

(12) Has the patient been informed of his/her rights both by word of mouth and in writing? Was the level of the patient's understanding recorded and is the information going to be repeated?

(13) Has the nearest relative been given the statutory information?

Figure 18.7 Check-list – section 2 (application for admission for assessment).

(14) If not, has the patient requested in writing that the information should not be given?

(15) Have Forms 14 and 15 been completed correctly?

(1) Is there an application by the approved social worker on Form 9 or an application by the nearest relative on Form 8?

(2) Have the social services been informed for the home circumstances report?

(3) Is the application signed?

(4) Is the date on which the applicant last saw the patient within 14 days of the date of the application?

(5) Is there a joint medical recommendation on Form 10, **or** are there separate medical recommendations on Form 11?

(6) Is one of the medical recommendations signed by a doctor who had previous acquaintance of the patient? If not does the application contain an explanation?

(7) Is one of the medical recommendations signed by a doctor approved for the purposes of section 12 of the Act?

(8) Have the recommending doctors examined the patient together or within 5 clear days of each other?

(9) Are the dates of both medical recommendations on or before the date of the signature of the application?

(10) Is the date of the admission within the period of 14 days beginning with the date of the later of the two medical recommendations?

(11) If both doctors work at the same hospital is the RMO aware of section 12(4)? (part- time doctor at the same hospital)

(12) Do the details on the medical recommendations correspond with the application form?

(13) Has the patient been given the statutory rights both by word of mouth and in writing? Was his level of understanding recorded and is a further attempt to be made?

(14) Has the nearest relative been given the statutory information? If not, has the patient requested in writing that this should not be given?

(15) Have Forms 14 and 15 been completed correctly?

Figure 18.8 Checklist – section 3 (admission for treatment).

Faxed documents

The fax machine is in increasing use and sometimes statutory documents are faxed between authorities. What is the legal situation?

Since the documents are the basis of the justification of the patient's detention, it is probably essential that the originals should be given to the managers, and that the approved social worker's application is based upon the original medical recommendations. Errors can occur in faxing, and it may be dangerous to rely upon a faxed document. The Home Office sometimes faxes documents to hospitals but the managers should insist that they receive the original documents as soon as possible from the Home Office. Similar provisions should take place when patients are transferred between hospitals. The receiving hospital should have the original documents relating to the patient's detention.

Questions and exercises

(1) What action should a nurse take when she discovers one of the statutory documents is incomplete? Would it make any difference if the detained patient had been admitted less than two weeks before?

(2) Following the detention of a patient under section 5(2) it was discovered that the doctor who signed the form was not the RMO nor was he designated under section 5(3). Seventy-two hours have now elapsed and the patient is informal. What action, if any, should be taken?

(3) A joint medical recommendation on Form 10 for section 3 admission has been jointly signed by the two doctors but one of the doctors has failed to write his name and address on the front

part of the form. Four weeks elapse before this error is noticed, is the patient validly detained? If not, what action can be taken assuming that the patient is still mentally disordered and requires to be treated in hospital, but would not be prepared to stay voluntarily?

Chapter 19   The mental health managers

The role of the managers in relation to their function in the Mental Health Act 1983 is considered in this chapter.

Definition

The first question to be answered is 'Who are they?' The definition of the managers is set out in Figure 19.1. Refer also to Chapter 24 of the Code of Practice.

Section 145 defines 'the managers' as:

(1) in relation to NHS hospitals – the district health authority or special health authority responsible for the administration of the hospital, or the NHS Trust Board;

(2) in relation to a Special Hospital – the Secretary of State;

(3) in relation to a mental nursing home registered in pursuance of the Nursing Homes Act 1975, the person or persons registered in respect of the home.

**Figure 19.1
Definition: mental
health managers.**

In the case of NHS hospitals therefore, the managers are members of the health authority or NHS Trust. All the functions of the managers can be delegated to officers except for those of hearing appeals against detention and reviewing the report recommending renewal. The latter functions cannot be delegated, but can be carried out by a committee of at least three members acting on the authority's behalf (section 23(4)).

In the case of NHS Trusts the managers are the non-executive directors of the trust, or their co-opted members.

Functions

Figure 19.2 sets out the functions of the managers under the Act and Regulations.

(1) To accept a patient and record admission Form 14 (Reg. 4.3).

(2) To give information to detained patients (section 132).

(3) To give information to the nearest relative unless the patient requests otherwise (section 132(4)).

(4) To give information to the nearest relative on the discharge of the patient unless the patient requests otherwise (section 133(1)).

(5) To inform the nearest relative of the continued detention of the patient after a report from the responsible medical officer (RMO) has been received (section 25(2)).

(6) To discharge the patient if appropriate (section 23(2)(b)).

(7) To refer the patient to a mental health review tribunal (MHRT) (section 68(1) and (2)).

(8) To transfer a patient (section 19(3), Section 19(1)(A), Reg. 7.2 and Reg. 7.3).

(9) To scrutinize and oversee the documentation and consider whether to give consent to rectification (section 15(1)).

(10) To oversee generally the care and treatment of the detained patient.

(11) In addition, the managers have overall responsibility for the care of all patients and therefore would also be responsible for the care of the informal patient.

Figure 19.2 Functions of the managers.

Duty to monitor the handling of complaints

In addition, though not set out in the Act, the managers have a duty to monitor the handling of complaints. As far as hospitals are concerned the Hospital Complaints Procedure Act 1985 applies and the members of the health authority or NHS Trust Board would be expected to have an overseeing role to ensure that the complaints procedure was operating effectively. Community health care was omitted from the Hospital Complaints Procedure Act but good practice and certainly the Patient's Charter would expect that complaints about community services should be handled in a similar way.

Discharge of patients

Discharge by the managers is considered in Chapter 9.

Check-list of functions

Figure 19.3 sets out a check-list for managers to follow in carrying out their functions under the Act and generally.

(1) Are the numbers of detained patients increasing or decreasing?

(2) Are there gaps in the time a patient is placed on sections 5(4), 5(2), 2, and 3 or are they all consecutive?

(3) How many records have to be rectified as a proportion of the total? What are the main errors? Who gives consent to the rectification? Is this ever refused?

(4) How often is a patient given statutory information during a period of detention? How is his understanding of this information reviewed?

(5) What proportion of appeals to managers or to the MHRT are successful?

(6) How often is a patient discharged from a section just before a managers' review or an MHRT?

(7) What monitoring exists to ensure a detained patient has given a valid consent to ECT or drugs after three months?

(8) How often is emergency treatment given to detained patients under section 62? Is there a requirement to complete a form?

(9) How often is seclusion used? What is the maximum time used for any one patient?

(10) Are the doors on wards with informal patients ever locked? How is this monitored?

(11) Do all the patients detained under section 3 have after-care plans? Are these arranged before discharge?

(12) How many detained patients are likely to be on leave of absence at any one time? How is the number recorded?

(13) What arrangements have been made with the general hospitals over the use of section 5(2)?

(14) How frequently is the Nurses' Holding Power used and on average how long does it last?

(15) Do the police constables bring patients straight to the hospital after arresting them in a place to which the public have access? What procedure exists?

(16) Is a distinction drawn between the handling of complaints of detained and non-detained patients?

(17) Do the managers ever challenge a doctor's recommendation for renewal?

(18) How often do managers visit wards and talk to patients (detained and non-detained) and staff?

(19) What criteria are used to judge whether the mental health services under their management are in a healthy state?

Figure 19.3 Check-list for managers.

(20) How frequently should an audit like this be carried out?

Question and exercises

(1) In what ways could you make most effective use of the Mental Health Act managers for the hospital?

(2) A friend has confided in you that he may be appointed as a Mental Health Act manager for the Trust. He asks you to explain the duties required.

(3) A patient has complained of being deprived of his day time clothes. You know that he has not received a reply from the designated complaints officer. What action could you take in relation to the managers?

Chapter 20   Mental Health Act Commission

The Mental Health Act Commission (MHAC) was set up under section 121 of the Mental Health Act 1983 as a special health authority. The Secretary of State is required to direct the MHAC to perform on his behalf specified functions.

What are its functions?

These are set out in section 121 of the Act and are shown in Figure 20.1.

(1)   To keep under review the operation of the Mental Health Act 1983 in respect of patients detained under the Act or patients liable to be detained under the Act.

(2)   To visit and interview (in private) patients detained under the Act in hospitals and mental nursing homes.

(3)   To investigate complaints which fall within the Commission's remit.

(4)   To review decisions to withhold the mail of patients detained in the Special Hospitals.

(5)   To appoint medical practitioners and others to give second opinions in cases where this is required by the Act.

(6)   To monitor the implementation of the Code of Practice and advise the Ministers on amendments.

(7)   To publish a biennial report

(8)   To offer advice to Ministers on matters falling within the Commission's remit.

Figure 20.1   Statutory functions of the Mental Health Act Commission.

What is the MHAC's function in relation to informal patients?

Section 121(4) gives to the Secretary of State the power (after consulting the MHAC and other bodies) to direct the MHAC to keep under review the care and treatment (or any aspect of the care and treatment) in hospitals and mental nursing homes of patients who are not liable to be detained under the Act. This provision has not however been implemented and there are considerable resource implications if it were to be.

What is the constitution of the MHAC?

The MHAC shall consist of such members as the Secretary of State may from time to time determine of whom one shall be chairman and one vice-chairman (Statutory Instrument 1983 No 892). There are about 90 members covering all the major professions involved with the care of the mentally disordered, psychiatrists, psychologists, nurses, social workers, lawyers, occupational therapists and lay members.

A Central Policy Committee is appointed by the Secretary of State from members of the MHAC which has the function of preparing the Code of Practice, the biennial report and any other function which the MHAC requires of it.

The MHAC is organized into visiting teams covering England and Wales. There are also national standing committees covering the topics set out in Figure 20.2.

Figure 20.2 National Standing Committees of the Mental Health Act Commission (topics).

(1) Research and information
(2) Visiting
(3) Learning disabilities
(4) Legal and parliamentary affairs
(5) Code of Practice
(6) Community care
(7) Race and culture
(8) Mentally disordered offenders
(9) Consent to treatment
(10) Complaints

The terms of reference of each committee are set out in Appendix 3 to the Fifth Biennial Report. It is vital that any concerns of nursing staff relating to these aspects of the care of detained patients should be sent to the Chief Executive of the Mental Health Act Commission for the attention of the appropriate committee since it is important that it should be made aware of concerns with the functioning of the Act or of the care of detained patients. The address can be found in the list of Useful Addresses. From November 1995 the Mental Health Act Commission has been reorganized and a new structure is to be created which will deal with policy issues.

What powers does it have?

The MHAC is given the power under the Act (section 120(4) and section 121(5)) and by Direction HC(83)19 of the Secretary of State for Social Services to visit and interview a detained patient and require the production of and inspect any records relating to the detention or treatment of any person who is or has been detained in a hospital or mental nursing home.

Section 129 makes it an offence to refuse to allow inspection of the premises, the visiting of patients, the production of documents, or otherwise to obstruct any person in the exercise of functions under the Act without reasonable cause.

Visiting

Commissioners attempt to visit each hospital or mental nursing home where patients are detained or liable to be detained at least once a year. Special Hospitals are visited much more frequently. Visits to regional secure units are made every six months. Visits are usually announced and information on the number of detained patients, sections they are under and details of consent to treatment provisions are requested from the managers before the anticipated visit. It is expected that the detained patients will be notified of a proposed visit and be given the opportunity to speak to the Commissioners (See Appendix II, Example J). The Commissioners will examine the statutory documents and the patients' records and review generally the workings and implementation of the Act.

The usual procedure is for the visiting commissioners to meet with the managers of the hospital initially and then to visit the wards and speak to the detained patients, looking at the records and documentation.

Unannounced visits are occasionally made if there is concern by the Commissioners over any issue relating to detained patients or the implementation of the Act. In the Fifth Biennial Report 1991–93 it is reported that there were only three unannounced visits out of 1089 visits to hospitals and three unannounced visit out of 34 to mental nursing homes.

Complaints

The Act (section 120(1)(b)) requires the Commission to investigate

'(i) any complaint made by a person in respect of a matter that occurred while he was detained under this Act in a hospital or mental nursing home and which he considers has not been satisfactorily dealt with by the managers of that hospital or mental nursing home; and

(ii) any other complaint as to the exercise of the powers or the discharge of the duties conferred or imposed by this Act in respect of a person who is or has been so detained.'

It would usually be expected therefore that any patient's complaint has already been made to the managers before the MHAC investigates it.

Staff can bring matters to the attention of the MHAC but it would be usually appropriate to them to draw the attention of management to the matter of concern first. Staff can refer patients' complaints as well as raise other issues relating to the Act. They would not however be able to raise issues relating to pay and conditions unless this had a direct bearing upon the exercise of powers and duties under the Act.

Recommendations of the enquiry into allegations at Ashworth Hospital chaired by Sir Louis Blom-Cooper recommended a change in the statutory function of the MHAC in relation to the investigation of complaints and recommended that it should have a monitoring rather than an investigatory role but could take direct referrals from the Secretary of State.

The complaints handled by the MHAC during 1991–1993 are shown in Figure 20.3 and show that the largest category of complaint related to medical treatment. This was also the highest category in the previous biennial report.

Figure 20.3 Complaints investigated by the Mental Health Act Commission Fifth Biennial Report 1991–93. *Note:* These percentages are indicative. They are taken from a bar chart and do not add up to 100%.

(a)	Offences against the person	11.0%
(b)	Medical care and services	12.0%
(c)	Medical treatment	15.0%
(d)	Nursing	6.0%
(e)	Other professional	7.0%
(f)	Domestic care	4.0%
(g)	Finance, benefits, property	4.0%
(h)	Deprivation of liberty	8.0%
(j)	Leave, parole etc.	5.5%
(k)	MHRTs	4.0%
(l)	Family matters	1.0%
(m)	Administration	2.0%
(n)	Local authority	0.8%
(o)	Social educational	0.2%
(p)	Ethnic etc.	0.8%
(q)	DoH, Home Office	0.4%
(r)	MHAC	0.2%
(s)	Others	2.2%

Procedure in handling complaints

The MHAC has complete discretion in how it investigates complaints. Sometimes it is appropriate for an issue to be taken up with management either at a local level or informally. Sometimes two Commissioners are sent to interview the patient and the relevant staff.

As a special health authority the Commission comes under the jurisdiction of the Health Service Commissioner (the Ombudsman) and complaints about the Commission could therefore be made to the Ombudsman (addresses for England and Wales are given in the list of Useful Addresses). These could pertain to its investigation of complaints or the carrying out of its other functions.

The Health Service Commissioner has powers to order the production of records and documents and to compel staff to give evidence before him. He can make recommendations for health authorities and NHS Trusts to apologize and/or to take remedial action and reform their procedures. He makes an annual report to Parliament and a select committee of the House of Commons reviews his activities and can initiate an enquiry into any matter he has investigated, summoning Board members and officers to the House of Commons to answer its questions. This is considered to be an effective weapon in securing compliance to the Health Service Commissioner's recommendations.

In 1994 the Wilson Report, *Being Heard* (1994, DoH) which made recommendations on a united procedure for the handling of complaints about hospital, community and primary health care services, recommended the same procedure for the handling of all complaints. This may lead to wider jurisdiction for the Health Service Commissioner to include complaints about clinical judgment.

The future of the Commission

An internal reorganization of the Commission was implemented in November 1995. It is aimed at increasing the number of detained patients seen by Commissioners and introduces different kinds of Commissioner. Some will only carry out visits; others will handle complaints and undertake a co-ordinating role.

Questions and exercises

(1) There is an announcement that the MHAC Commissioners are due to visit the hospital the following month, what action would you take in relation to:

       (a) detained patients,

       (b) detained patients who are on section 17 leave,

       (c) informal patients,

       (d) the staff on the ward and

       (e) the records?

(2)   In what ways could you make most use of a visit by the Commissioners?

(3)   You are aware that a patient has complained to the hospital managers of an assault by a member of staff but has had no reply, what duties and rights would you have in relation to the MHAC?

(4)   What is the difference in function/powers and procedures of the Mental Health Act Commission compared with those of the Health Service Commissioner?

Chapter 21

Offences under the Act and staff protection against court action by the patient

All professionals are liable to both criminal and civil proceedings as a result of their work. The care of the mentally disordered is no exception. The patients/clients are vulnerable and require a high standard of care and protection. The Mental Health Acts 1959 and 1983 therefore provide a number of offences related to the care of the detained patients and these are set out below. For the non-detained patient however the ordinary criminal laws relating to offences against the person, theft, fraud and criminal damage all provide the protection available to the ordinary citizen. These laws also apply to the protection of the detained patient. Staff could be prosecuted under these laws.

Similarly the staff face the possibility of civil action in relation to their work such as actions for negligence, trespass to the person, false imprisonment and breach of statutory duty. Usually the civil action is brought by the injured person to obtain damages and therefore it is more likely to be directed against the employer than the staff on the basis of its vicarious liability for the wrongful actions of its employees. Since 1990 the health service body, under arrangements agreed with the Department of Health and set out in circular HC(89)34 which effectively replaces HM(54)32, has accepted liability for the negligent acts of doctors and dentists who had in the past been sued personally.

In addition the Act recognizes that staff are vulnerable because in exceptional circumstances some mentally disordered patients may be more likely to complain as a result of their mental condition. Persons who have recourse to the courts to an exceptional degree are known as vexatious litigants (see Glossary). The Act makes provisions for certain hurdles to be passed before a court action (whether civil or criminal) can proceed against a member of staff. These provisions are set out in section 139 and are discussed below.

Criminal offences in the Act

Certain sections in the Act make it a criminal offence to fail to comply with its provisions. These are set out in Part IX of the Act:

Section 126 – forgery and false statements.
Section 127 – ill-treatment of patients.
Section 128 – assisting patients to absent themselves without leave.
Section 129 – obstruction to those carrying out duties under the Act.

Section 130 enables the local authority to bring a prosecution for such offences which are discussed below in detail.

Forgery and false statements

Section 126 makes it an offence for a person to have in his custody or control without lawful authority or excuse any document to which the subsection applies or which he knows or believes to be false. The section also covers any document so closely resembling one of these documents as to be calculated to deceive. The documents covered are set out in Figure 21.1.

Documents covered by section 126

- an application under Part II
- a medical recommendation or report
- any other document required or authorized to be made for any purposes under the Act

Offences – false entries
Section 126(4) makes it an offence:

- wilfully to make a false entry or statement in any application, recommendation, report, record or other document required or authorized to be made for any purposes under the Act, **or**
- with intent to deceive, to make use of any such entry or statement which he knows to be false.

Penalties
For an offence under this section

- on summary conviction (i.e. before the magistrates) up to six months imprisonment or a fine not exceeding the statutory maximum, £5000, or both
- on conviction on indictment (i.e. in the crown court) imprisonment up to two years or to a fine of any amount or both.

Figure 21.1 Elements of section 126 (forgery and false statements).

Ill-treatment of patients

This is covered in section 127, set out in Figure 21.2.

Persons covered
Any person who

- is an officer on the staff of, or
- otherwise employed in, or
- is one of the managers of

a hospital or mental nursing home.

Offences
Section 127(1) makes it an offence

(a)   to ill-treat or wilfully to neglect a patient for the time being receiving treatment for mental disorder as an in-patient in that hospital or home; **or**

(b)   to ill-treat or wilfully to neglect, on the premises of which the hospital or home forms part, a patient for the time being receiving such treatment there as an out-patient.

Figure 21.2   Elements of section 127(1) (ill-treatment of patients).

Penalties
These are the same as for section 126 (see Figure 21.1).

It is also an offence for any individual to ill-treat or wilfully neglect a mentally disordered patient who is for the time being subject to his guardianship under the Act or otherwise in his custody or care (whether by virtue of any legal or moral obligation or otherwise) (section 127(2)).

The consent of the Director of Public Prosecutions is required before proceedings can be instituted for these offences.

Assisting patients to absent themselves without leave

This is summarized in Figure 21.3.

Offences
Section 128 provides for the following to have committed offences:

- Any person who induces or knowingly assists another person who is liable to be detained in a hospital within the meaning of Part II of the Act or is subject to guardianship to absent himself without leave.

● Any person who induces or knowingly assists another person who is in legal custody by virtue of section 137 to escape from custody.

● Any person who knowingly harbours a patient who is absent without leave or is otherwise at large and liable to be retaken under the Act or gives him assistance with intent to prevent, hinder or interfere with his being taken into custody or returned to the hospital or other place where he ought to be.

Penalties

These are the same as for sections 126 and 127 (see Figure 21.1).

Figure 21.3 Offences under section 128 (assisting with absence without leave).

Obstruction

Section 129 creates several offences which are set out in Figure 21.4.

Person/offences covered

Any person who without reasonable cause:

● refuses to allow the inspection of any premises; or
● refuses to allow the visiting, interviewing or examination of any person by a person authorized in that behalf or under the Act; or
● refuses to produce for the inspection of any person so authorized any document or record the production of which is duly required by him; or
● otherwise obstructs any such person in the exercise of his functions, or
● insists on being present when required to withdraw by a person authorized by or under the Act to interview or examine a person in private

is guilty of an offence.

Penalties

On summary conviction to imprisonment up to three months or to a fine not exceeding level 4 (£2500) on the standard scale or to both.

Figure 21.4 Elements of section 129 (obstruction).

Prosecution by local social services authority

Section 130 enables the local social services authority to institute proceedings for any offence but the consent of the Director of Public Prosecutions is still required if this is laid down in the Act.

when the permitted visiting time is ended. The respondent was accordingly acting in pursuance of the 1959 Act when the incident complained of occurred and before civil or criminal proceedings for assault could properly be brought against him, the leave of the High Court should have been sought and obtained.'

Lord Edmund Davies quoted with approval the words of Lord Widgery CJ in his judgment in the Divisional Court:

'In my judgment where a male nurse is on duty and exercising his function of controlling patients in the hospital, acts done in pursuance of such control or purportedly in pursuance of such control are acts within the scope of section 141 and are thus protected by the section.'

Following this decision it is difficult to think of any action done in relation to a detained patient which will not be caught by this wide interpretation.

Protection given to staff in relation to detained patients in comparison with informal patients

There is a large gulf between the protection afforded to staff in relation to those detained under the Act and in relation to those who are informal patients. Acts done in relation to informal patients like ushering a patient back to his ward after visiting would not come within the protection provided by section 139. If on the other hand an informal patient were to be detained under section 5(2) or section 5(4) or be subject to the consent to treatment provisions of section 57 (brain surgery or hormonal implants) and wished to bring a civil or criminal action in relation to that activity, the protection afforded by section 139 would then apply.

The section therefore places a hurdle in the way of the detained patient but not the informal patient, a distinction which cannot necessarily be justified.

Judicial review

An application can be made to court for the review of administrative judicial decisions. An example is the case of *R* v. *Hallstrom, ex parte W* (1985). This was an application, not to claim damages against a doctor, but to seek an inquiry into the decision made as to whether there had been an excess of jurisdiction or not. The patient in this case had been admitted to the hospital under section 3 and released the next day under section 17 subject to conditions as to treatment. The Mental Health Review Tribunal refused her application for discharge.

The Queen's Bench hearing (Mr. Justice McCullough) decided that section 3 did not authorize a nominal period of detention for a time when no necessary treatment was required to be given, and that since the doctors considered that she should receive treatment while living in the hostel, and did not consider that treatment as an in-patient was appropriate, their recommendations for her admission for treatment overnight, purportedly in accordance with section 3, were unlawful.

Liability of the health authority or NHS Trust

Detained patients

The protection afforded to a potential defendant by section 139(1) and (2) does not apply to the Secretary of State or health authority (section 139(4)). It is not necessary therefore for the applicant to apply to a High Court Judge or Director of Public Prosecution for leave to bring the action.

Nor is it necessary to show the act was done in bad faith or without reasonable care. However in practice the health authority will not be held vicariously liable for its employees unless the employees have been negligent or committed a tortious act. In practice therefore the common law will provide a defence for the health authority comparable with the statutory defence against personal liability in relation to allegations relating to detained patients.

Informal patients

As far as an action relating to informal patients is concerned, the health authority or NHS Trust is in the same position as the individual employee or professional. Once a duty of care is established in relation to the patient, the individual person will be liable for any breach of duty which causes harm to the patient and the health authority or Trust is vicariously liable for its employees. If the legal action is based on negligence then damage suffered by the patient must be established. If the action is based on trespass to the person or false imprisonment then no specific harm need be proved, i.e. it is actionable *per se.*

Questions and exercises

(1) A former detained patient has threatened to sue a registered nurse for the mentally ill for neglect during her stay in hospital. What protection does the nurse have? What steps should she take?

(2)   A medical records officer noticed that the GP who wrote one of the medical recommendations for admission under section 3 had signed the form but had not completed his full name and address. She therefore completed it for him. The patient had already been admitted for three weeks. Is this an offence under the Act?

(3)   Mental Health Act Commissioners visit a ward to interview a detained patient but the ward sister, believing the patient is too ill to see them refuses entry. Is this an offence under the act?

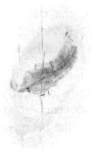

Chapter 22   Conclusion

The registered nurse is personally and professionally accountable for her care of the patient and for ensuring that she complies
with the law. Ignorance of the law is no defence and the nurse
must therefore ensure that she is fully conversant with the
details of the law relating to both the detained and the informal
mentally disturbed patient. She must be familiar with the
sources of information and guidance available to her. Ultimately
it is her responsibility to ensure that she knows the legal status
of the patient and the implications which flow from that. She
should be aware of the lengths of permissible detention and
ensure that appropriate action is taken when necessary. She
should therefore familiarize herself with the patient's records
which should set out

- the details of the admission,
- section 17 leave permission,
- the date medication commenced (significant for the com-
  mencement of section 58 provisions in relation to medication), and
- the dates on which an application to the Mental Health
  Review Tribunal can be made by the patient, or
- must be made by the managers.

She should also ensure that she takes steps to refresh her
knowledge of the law and keep up-to-date with changes. The
Government announced in November 1994 that amendments
would be made to the Mental Health Act 1983 in the forth-
coming parliamentary session. This was enacted in 1995 and
included not only the introduction of a community supervision
order, but also an amendment to the current provision whereby
the section ends for non-restricted patients if the patient is
absent without leave for longer than 28 days. These statutory
changes are contained in the Mental Health (Patients in the
Community) Act 1995. It may be that this legislation will be
followed by a review of all the provisions of the Mental Health
Act. The nurse should ensure that she has an input into the

discussion which takes place over the future laws relating to the mentally disordered patient. Only if she is confident in her knowledge of the present law, and understands its strengths and weaknesses in relation to the care of the patient, can she play an informed part in this important debate which will take us into the 21st century.

Glossary

Definitions of certain terms and more details of some of the cases referred to in the text are given below.

Bolam Test

A health professional is not negligent if he adopts a practice which a responsible body of skilled medical men would accept as proper.

Discharge from section

Removal from legal detention under the Mental Health Act. This changes the status of a patient from that of compulsory detention to 'informal' or voluntary status.
Note that this does not necessarily mean discharge from hospital care.

Disposals

Choices open to court for care of patients.

Ex parte

A term occurring in the title of cases concerning judicial review meaning 'on behalf of' and identifying the person affected by the administrative decision which is being reviewed by the court and who is bringing the action.

F v. West Berkshire Health Authority

This case was concerned with the sterilization of a severely mentally handicapped woman who was incapable of giving a valid consent. The House of Lords stated that if the doctors acted in her best interests and followed the accepted approved practice of a reasonable doctor they would not be acting unlawfully. This ruling would also apply to the work of a nurse. In serious and non-urgent cases such as sterilization the court felt, however, that the matter should be brought to the court first.

Gillick competence

The House of Lords held that a child of under 16 years with sufficient maturity to understand the implications of a decision could give a valid consent to treatment.

Informal status

That of a person who is admitted to hospital without the formalities of the Mental Health Act or comparable legislation.

Legal detention

Being held under a section of the Mental Health Act or comparable legislation.

Managers	In relation to NHS hospitals: the district health authority or special health authority responsible for the administration of the hospital or the NHS Trust Board. In relation to Special Hospitals: the Secretary of State. In relation to mental nursing homes registered in pursuance of the Nursing Homes Act 1975: the person or persons registered.
M'Naghten rules	These were laid down in the 19th century. In the ruling 'not guilty by reason of insanity', insanity is defined by the courts using these rules. It is necessary to show:

'that, at the time of committing the act, the party accused was labouring under such a defect of reason, from disease of the mind, as not to know the nature and quality of the act he was doing, or, if he did know it, that he did not know that what he was doing was wrong.'

Medical treatment	The wide definition includes nursing, care, habilitation and rehabilitation under medical supervision.
Nearest relative	The person likely to be closest to the patient. Defined in Section 26 of the Act. See Figure 7.1.
Pro re nata (PRN)	As necessary/as required. Usually applied to medication.
Purchaser	The body paying for medical treatment.
R or Rex or Regina v.	This stands for 'the Crown versus' in giving the title of a criminal case or one concerning judicial review.
R v. Ealing District Health Authority, ex parte Fox	A restricted patient was given a conditional discharge by a Mental Health Review Tribunal, the discharge being deferred until the Tribunal was satisfied that a consultant psychiatrist was appointed to act as the patient's responsible medical officer (RMO). Neither the consultant forensic psychiatrist nor the consultant general psychiatrist for the patient's home were prepared to act as the RMO for the patient. The general manager of the health authority accordingly wrote to the patient. The patient applied to the court seeking a judicial review of the health authority's failure to provide a RMO in fulfilment of its duty to provide aftercare under section 117. The judge held that the health authority had erred in law in not attempting with all reasonable expedition and diligence to make arrangements so as to enable the patient to comply with the conditions laid down by the Tribunal. The court did not however make an order for mandamus which would have compelled the health authority to provide psychiatric supervision in the community for the patient.
R v. Hallstrom, ex parte W	Miss W. had a long history of chronic schizophrenic illness and had been admitted to hospital many times. She was admitted under Section

3 on 24 July 1984 and the day after admission was given Section 17 leave of absence by her RMO. She challenged the validity of the detention and the judge held that it had been shown for the purposes of section 3 that the patient's mental condition required detention in hospital. In a case heard at the same time (*R. v. Gardner, ex parte L*) the issue in question was the renewal of detention after the first six months' detention under section 3. The court held that, if the patient's mental condition did not require him to be detained in hospital, it was not permissible to recall a patient who was on section 17 leave to hospital in order to renew the section.

Re
This is Latin for 'about'. It is used to retain anonymity of persons reported in legal cases.

Re T (consent to medical treatment: adult patient)
The patient was the daughter of a Jehovah's Witness mother and she refused to have a blood transfusion. The court emphasized the right of the adult mentally competent patient to refuse to consent to even life saving treatment but also the duty of the doctor to ensure that the refusal was valid. In that case the judge hearing the case in the High Court considered that the will of the patient had been overborne by the influence of the mother and when she refused to give consent to a blood transfusion she had been lulled into a false sense of security by the staff who at that stage did not realize that a blood transfusion might become essential. The Court of Appeal upheld the decision of the judge and stated that:

'In all cases doctors need to consider what is the true scope and basis of the refusal. Was it intended to apply in the circumstances which have arisen? Was it based upon assumptions which in the event have not been realized? A refusal is only effective within its true scope and is vitiated if it is based upon false assumptions.'

Responsible Medical Officer (RMO)
A registered medical practitioner in charge of the treatment of patients under section 2 or section 3.

Second opinion appointed doctor
A registered medical practitioner appointed by the MHAC to provide an independent opinion for the purposes of Part IV, Consent to Treatment.

Section 12 approved doctor
Lists of doctors approved as having special experience in the diagnosis or treatment of mental disorder are kept by regional branches of the NHSME or by Health Authorities in Wales. That such approved doctors are available is required by section 12 of the Act, and they are known colloquially as 'section 12 approved doctors'.

Sidaway case
In this case the House of Lords stated that there was not in English law a concept of informed consent. There was however a duty upon the

doctor to follow the Bolam Test in giving information to the patient, i.e. the doctor must follow the standard of the reasonable professional.

Statutory   Required or permitted by a written law passed by a legislative body, e.g. an Act of Parliament.

Statutory duty   Duty required by a written law passed by a legislative body, e.g. an Act of Parliament.

Statutory Instrument (SI)   Delegated legislation passed not by Parliament but drafted by the relevant state department under powers given in an Act of Parliament. Statutory Rules or Regulations are usually drafted as Statutory Instruments and placed before the Houses of Parliament.

Therapeutic privilege   The Law recognizes the doctor's right to withhold information where that is in the best interests of the patient. This is known as 'therapeutic privilege' and should be exercised only in exceptional circumstances.

Top-slicing   Funding kept centrally to meet specific priorities/services.

Vexatious litigants   Persons who have recourse to the courts to an exceptional degree and who need to apply to the Court for leave to start a legal action.

Table of Cases

B *v.* Croydon Health Authority (1994) (The Times Law Report 1 Dec. 1994) 61–2, 67

Black *v.* Forsey (1988) 90

D'Souza *v.* The Director of Public Prosecutions (1992) 4 All ER 1995 89

F *v.* West Berkshire Health Authority (1989) .. 59, 60, 68, 70, 90, 150

Gillick *v.* West Norfolk and Wisbech Area Health Authority (1985) 69

Poutney *v.* Griffiths (1975) 2 All ER 881 144–5

R *v.* Ealing District Health Authority, ex parte Fox (1993) .. 116, 151

R *v.* Hallstrom, ex parte W and R *v.* Gardner, ex parte L (1985) 87, 145, 151–2

R *v.* Kirklees Metropolitan Borough Council, ex parte C (1993) ... 22

R *v.* Mental Health Act Commission, ex parte W (1988) 63

Re C (adult: refusal of medical treatment) (1994) 68, 70

Re T (consent to medical treatment: adult patient) (1992) 69, 152

Re W (a minor) (medical treatment) (1992) 69

Sidaway *v.* Board of Governors of Bethlem Royal Hospital (1985) 48, 152

W *v.* L (1974) 13–14

See also Glossary

Table of Statutes and Statutory Instruments

Table of Statutes

Access to Health Records Act 1990 49
Children Act 1989 .... 53, 69
Criminal Procedure (Insanity) Act 1964 .... 34, 35, 36, 43
Criminal Procedure (Insanity and Unfitness to Plead) Act 1991
.... 34, 35
Family Law Reform Act 1969 69
Health Service Act 1995 120
Hospital Complaints Procedure Act 1985 .... 48, 130
Immigration Act 1971 .... 42, 43
Magistrates Courts Act 1980 42
Mental Health Act 1959 .... 52, 139, 143, 144, 145
Mental Health Act 1983
.... 1–4, 33, 36, 52, 59, 106, 110, 118, 133, 139, 148, 157–67
Mental Health (Patients in the Community) Act 1995
.... 4, 83, 87, 117, 119, 120, 148, 168–72
Mental Health (Scotland) Act 1984 90
National Assistance Act 1948 96
National Health Service Act 1977 96
National Health Service and Community Care Act 1990 .... 115, 117
Nurses, Midwives and Health Visitors Act 1979 27
Nursing Homes Act 1975 .... 129, 151
Police and Criminal Evidence Act 1984 .... 48, 59, 89, 93, 98
Sexual Offences Act 1956 53

Table of Statutory Instruments

The Mental Health (Nurses) Order 1983 (SI 1983 No. 891) (and
    amending order) (SI 1993 No. 2155) 27
The Mental Health Review Tribunal Rules 1983 (SI 1983 No. 942)
    .... 49, 74, 75, 77, 78
Mental Health Act Commission, Establishment and Constitution 1983
    (SI 1983 No. 892) 134
The Mental Health (Hospital, Guardianship and Consent to Treatment)
    Regulations 1983 (SI 1983 No. 893) 57, 100, 102, 107, 108

Extracts from the Mental Health Act 1983

Note Square brackets and text in italic print indicate paraphrases of the statutory provisions.

Part I Application of Act

Section 1

Definition of Mental Disorder [*see Chapter 3*]

Section 1(3) *Exclusions from the definition of mental disorder*

Nothing in subsection (2) above shall be construed as implying that a person may be dealt with under this Act as suffering from mental disorder, or from any form of mental disorder described in this section, by reason only of promiscuity or other immoral conduct, sexual deviancy or dependence on alcohol or drugs.

Part II Compulsory Admission to Hospital and Guardianship

Section 2

Admission for assessment

Section 2(1)

A patient may be admitted to a hospital and detained there for a period allowed by subsection (4) below in pursuance of an application (in this Act referred to as "an application for admission for assessment") made in accordance with subsections (2) and (3) below.

Section 2(2)

An application for admission for assessment may be made in respect of a patient on the grounds that —
(a) he is suffering from mental disorder of a nature or degree which warrants the detention of the patient in a hospital for assessment (or for assessment followed by medical treatment) for at least a limited period; and
(b) he ought to be so detained in the interests of his own health or safety or with a view to the protection of other persons.

Section 2(3)

An application for admission for assessment shall be founded on the written recommendations in the prescribed form of two registered medical practitioners, including in each case a statement that in the opinion of the practitioner the conditions set out in subsection (2) above are complied with.

Section 2(4)

Subject to the provisions of section 29(4) below, a patient admitted to hospital in pursuance of an application for admission for assessment may be detained for a period not exceeding 28 days beginning with the day on which he was admitted, but shall not be detained after the expiration of that period unless before it has expired he has become liable to be detained by virtue of a subsequent application, order or direction under the following provisions of this Act.

Section 3 | **Admission for treatment**

Section 3(1) | A patient may be admitted to a hospital and detained there for the period allowed by the following provisions of this Act in pursuance of an application (in this Act referred to as "an application for admission for treatment") made in accordance with this section.

Section 3(2) | An application for admission for treatment may be made in respect of a patient on the grounds that —

(a) he is suffering from mental illness, severe mental impairment, psychopathic disorder or mental impairment and his mental disorder is of a nature or degree which makes it appropriate for him to receive medical treatment in a hospital; and

(b) in the case of psychopathic disorder or mental impairment, such treatment is likely to alleviate or prevent a deterioration of his condition; and

(c) it is necessary for the health or safety of the patient or for the protection of other persons that he should receive such treatment and it cannot be provided unless he is detained under this section.

Section 3(3) | An application for admission for treatment shall be founded on the written recommendations in the prescribed form of two registered medical practitioners, including in each case a statement that in the opinion of the practitioner the conditions set out in subsection (2) above are complied with; and each such recommendation shall include —

(a) such particulars as may be prescribed of the grounds for that opinion so far as it relates to the conditions set out in paragraphs (a) and (b) of that subsection; and

(b) a statement of the reasons for that opinion so far as it relates to the conditions set out in paragraph (c) of that subsection, specifying whether other methods of dealing with the patient are available and, if so, why they are not appropriate.

Section 4 | **Admission for assessment in cases of emergency**

Section 4(1) | In any case of urgent necessity, an application for admission for assessment may be made in respect of a patient in accordance with the following provisions of this section, and any application so made is in this Act referred to as "an emergency application".

Section 4(2) | An emergency application may be made either by an approved social worker or by the nearest relative of the patient; and every such application shall include a statement that it is of urgent necessity for the patient to be admitted and detained under section 2 above, and that compliance with the provisions of this Part of this Act relating to applications under that section would involve undesirable delay.

Section 4(3)

An emergency application shall be sufficient in the first instance if founded on one of the medical recommendations required by section 2 above, given, if practicable, by a practitioner who has previous acquaintance with the patient and otherwise complying with the requirements of section 12 below so far as applicable to a single recommendation, and verifying the statement referred to in subsection (2) above.

Section 4(4)

An emergency application shall cease to have effect on the expiration of a period of 72 hours from the time when the patient is admitted to the hospital unless —
(a) the second medical recommendation required by section 2 above is given and received by the managers within that period; and
(b) that recommendation and the recommendation referred to in subsection (3) above together comply with all the requirements of section 12 below (other than the requirement as to the time of signature of the second recommendation).

Section 5

Application in respect of patient already in hospital

Section 5(1)

An application for the admission of a patient to a hospital may be made under this Part of this Act notwithstanding that the patient is already an in-patient in that hospital or, in the case of an application for admission for treatment that the patient is for the time being liable to be detained in the hospital in pursuance of an application for admission for assessment; and where an application is so made the patient shall be treated for the purpose of this Part of this Act as if he had been admitted to the hospital at the time when that application was received by the managers.

Section 5(2)

If, in the case of a patient who is an in-patient in a hospital, it appears to the registered medical practitioner in charge of the treatment of the patient that an application ought to be made under this Part of this Act for the admission of the patient to hospital, he may furnish to the managers a report in writing to that effect; and in any such case the patient may be detained in the hospital for a period of 72 hours from the time when the report is so furnished.

Section 5(3)

The registered medical practitioner in charge of the treatment of a patient in a hospital may nominate one (but not more than one) other registered medical practitioner on the staff of that hospital to act for him under subsection (2) above in his absence.

Section 5(4) *Nurse's Holding Power*

If, in the case of a patient who is receiving treatment for mental disorder as an in-patient in a hospital, it appears to a nurse of the prescribed class —
(a) that the patient is suffering from mental disorder to such a degree

that it is necessary for his health or safety or for the protection of others for him to be immediately restrained from leaving the hospital; and

(b) that it is not practicable to secure the immediate attendance of a practitioner for the purpose of furnishing a report under subsection (2) above,

the nurse may record that fact in writing; and in that event the patient may be detained in the hospital for a period of six hours from the time when that fact is so recorded or until the earlier arrival at the place where the patient is detained of a practitioner having the power to furnish a report under that subsection.

Section 5(5)   A record made under subsection (4) above shall be delivered by the nurse (or by a person authorised by the nurse in that behalf) to the managers of the hospital as soon as possible after it is made; and where a record is made under that subsection the period mentioned in subsection (2) [*72 hours*] shall begin at the time it is made.

Section 5(6)   The reference in subsection (1) above to an in-patient does not include an in-patient who is liable to be detained in pursuance of an application under this Part of this Act and the references in subsections (2) and (4) above do not include an in-patient who is liable to be detained in a hospital under this Part of this Act.

Section 12   **General provisions as to medical recommendations**

Section 12(1)   The recommendations required for the purposes of an application for the admission of a patient under this Part of this Act (in this Act referred to as "medical recommendations") shall be signed on or before the date of the application, and shall be given by practitioners who have personally examined the patient either together or separately, but where they have examined the patient separately not more than five days must have elapsed between the days on which the separate examinations took place.

Section 12(3)   Subject to subsection (4) below, where the application is for the admission of the patient to a hospital which is not a mental nursing home, one (but not more than one) of the medical recommendations may be given by a practitioner on the staff of that hospital, except where the patient [*will be a private patient*].

Section 12(4) *Factors allowing two doctors from the same hospital to make recommendations on the same patient*

(a) compliance with [*the requirement for only one doctor to be on the staff of the hospital*] would result in delay involving serious risk to the health or safety of the patient; and

(b) one of the practitioners giving the recommendations works at the hospital for less than half of the time which he is bound by contract to devote to work in the health service; and

(c) where one of those practitioners is a consultant, the other does not work (whether at the hospital or elsewhere) in a grade in which he is under that consultant's directions.

Section 12(5) *Persons prohibited from making the medical recommendation*

A medical recommendation for the purposes of an application for the admission of a patient under this Part of this Act shall not be given by —

(a) the applicant;

(b) a partner of the applicant or of a practitioner by whom another medical recommendation is given for the purposes of the same application;

(c) a person employed as an assistant by the applicant or by any such practitioner;

(d) a person who receives or has an interest in the receipt of any payments made on account of the maintenance of the patient; or

(e) except as provided by subsection (3) or (4) above, a practitioner on the staff of the hospital to which the patient is to be admitted,

or by the husband, wife, father, father-in-law, mother, mother-in-law, son, son-in-law, daughter, daughter-in-law, brother, brother-in-law, sister or sister-in-law of the patient, or of any person mentioned in paragraphs (a) to (e) above, or of a practitioner by whom another medical recommendation is given for the purposes of the same application.

Section 15

Rectification of applications and recommendations

Section 15(1)

If within the period of 14 days beginning with the day on which a patient has been admitted to a hospital in pursuance of an application for admission for assessment or for treatment the application, or any medical recommendation given for the purposes of the application, is found to be in any respect incorrect or defective, the application or recommendation may, within that period and with the consent of the managers of the hospital, be amended by the person by whom it was signed; and upon such amendment being made the application or recommendation shall have effect and shall be deemed to have had effect as if it had been originally made as so amended.

Section 15(2) *Rectification of documents if one of the medical recommendations is found to be insufficient*

...if [*within 14 days of the patient being admitted for assessment or treatment*] it appears to the managers of the hospital that one of the two medical recommendations on which the application for the admission of the patient is founded is insufficient to warrant the detention of the patient in pursuance of the application, they may, within that period, give notice in writing to that effect to the applicant; and ... that recommendation shall be disregarded, but the application shall be, and shall be deemed always to have been, sufficient if —

(a) a fresh medical recommendation complying with the relevant provisions of this Part of this Act (other than the provisions relating to the time of signature and the interval between examinations) is furnished to the managers within that period; and

(b) that recommendation, and the other recommendation on which the application is founded, together comply with those provisions.

Section 16

Reclassification of patients

Section 16(1)

If in the case of a patient who is for the time being detained in a hospital in pursuance of an application for admission for treatment, or subject to guardianship in pursuance of a guardianship application, it appears to the appropriate medical officer that the patient is suffering from a form of mental disorder other than the form or forms specified in the application, he may furnish to the managers of the hospital, or to the guardian, as the case may be, a report to that effect; and where a report is so furnished, the application shall have effect as if that other form of mental disorder were specified in it.

Section 17

Leave of absence from hospital [*with consent*]

Section 17(1)

The responsible medical officer may grant to any patient who is for the time being liable to be detained in a hospital under this Part of this Act leave to be absent from the hospital subject to such conditions (if any) as that officer considers necessary in the interests of the patient or for the protection of other persons.

Section 17(2)

Leave of absence may be granted to a patient under this section either indefinitely or on specified occasions or for any specified period; and where leave is so granted for a specified period, that period may be extended by further leave granted in the absence of the patient.

Section 17(3)

Where it appears to the responsible medical officer that it is necessary so to do in the interests of the patient or for the protection of other persons, he may, upon granting leave of absence under this section, direct that the patient remain in custody during his absence; and where leave of absence is so granted the patient may be kept in the custody of any officer on the staff of the hospital, or any other person authorised in writing by the managers of the hospital or, if the patient is required in accordance with conditions imposed on the grant of leave of absence to reside in another hospital, of any officer on the staff of that other hospital.

Section 17(4)

In any case where a patient is absent from a hospital in pursuance of leave of absence granted under this section, and it appears to the responsible medical officer that it is necessary so to do in the interests of the patient's health or safety or for the protection of other persons, that officer may, subject to subsection (5) below, by notice in writing given to the patient or to the person for the time being in charge of the patient, revoke the leave of absence and recall the patient to the hospital.

Section 17(5)

A patient to whom leave of absence is granted under this section shall not be recalled under subsection (4) above after he has ceased to be liable to be detained under this Part of this Act; and without prejudice to any other provision of this Part of this Act any such patient shall cease to be so liable at the expiration of the period of six months beginning with the first day of his absence on leave unless either —

(a) he has returned to the hospital, or has been transferred to another hospital under the following provisions of this Act, before the expiration of that period; or

(b) he is absent without leave at the expiration of that period.

Section 18   **Return and readmission of patients absent without leave**

Section 19   **Transfer of patients**

Section 20   **Duration of authority**

Section 20(3)   Within the period of two months ending on the day on which a patient who is liable to be detained in pursuance of an application for admission for treatment would cease under this section to be so liable in default of the renewal of the authority for his detention, it shall be the duty of the responsible medical officer —

(a) to examine the patient; and

(b) if it appears to him that the conditions set out in subsection (4) below are satisfied, to furnish to the managers of the hospital where the patient is detained a report to that effect in the prescribed form;

and where such a report is furnished in respect of a patient, the managers shall, unless they discharge the patient, cause him to be informed.

Section 20(4)   The conditions referred to in subsection (3) above are that —

(a) the patient is suffering from mental illness, severe mental impairment, psychopathic disorder or mental impairment, and his mental disorder is of a nature or degree which makes it appropriate for him to receive medical treatment in a hospital; and

(b) such treatment is likely to alleviate or prevent a deterioration of his condition; and

(c) it is necessary for the health or safety of the patient or for the protection of other persons that he should receive such treatment and that it cannot be provided unless he continues to be detained.

Part III Patients Concerned in Criminal Proceedings or Under Sentence

Section 35   **Remand to hospital for report on accused's mental condition**

Section 36   **Remand of accused person to hospital for treatment**

Section 37   Hospital Order or Guardianship with or without restriction order under Section 41 (mentally disordered offenders)

Section 38   **Interim hospital orders**

Section 41   **Power of higher courts to restrict discharge from hospital** [*restriction orders*]

Section 47   **Removal to hospital of persons serving sentences of imprisonment, etc.**

Section 48   **Removal to hospital of other prisoners**

Part IV Consent to Treatment

Section 57

Treatment requiring consent and a second opinion.

Section 57(1)

This section applies to the following forms of medical treatment for mental disorder —
(a) any surgical operation for destroying brain tissue or for destroying the functioning of brain tissue; and
(b) such other forms of treatment as may be specified for the purposes of this section by regulations made by the Secretary of State.

Section 57(2)

Subject to section 62 below, a patient shall not be given any form of treatment to which this section applies unless he has consented to it and —
(a) a registered medical practitioner appointed for the purposes of this Part of this Act by the Secretary of State (not being the responsible medical officer) and two other persons appointed for the purposes of this paragraph by the Secretary of State (not being registered medical practitioners) have certified in writing that the patient is capable of understanding the nature, purpose and likely effects of the treatment in question and has consented to it; and
(b) the registered medical practitioner referred to in paragraph (a) above has certified in writing that, having regard to the likelihood of the treatment alleviating or preventing a deterioration of the patient's condition, the treatment should be given.

Section 57(3)

Before giving a certificate under subsection (2)(b) above the registered medical practitioner concerned shall consult two other persons who have been professionally concerned with the patient's medical treatment, and of those persons one shall be a nurse and the other shall be neither a nurse nor a registered medical practitioner.

Section 57(4)

Before making any regulations for the purpose of this section the Secretary of State shall consult such bodies as appear to him to be concerned.

Section 58

Treatment requiring consent or a second opinion.

Section 58(1)

This section applies to the following forms of medical treatment for mental disorder —
(a) such forms of treatment as may be specified for the purposes of this section by regulations made by the Secretary of State;
(b) the administration of medicine to a patient by any means (not being a form of treatment specified under paragraph (a) above or section 57 above) at any time during a period for which he is liable to be detained as a patient to whom this Part of this Act applies if three months or more have elapsed since the first occasion in that period when medicine was administered to him by any means for his mental disorder.

Section 58(2)	The Secretary of State may by order vary the length of the period mentioned in subsection (1)(b) above.

Section 58(3)
Subject to section 62 below [*urgent treatment to be given compulsorily*], a patient shall not be given any form of treatment to which this section applies unless —
(a) he has consented to that treatment and either the responsible medical officer or a registered medical practitioner appointed for the purposes of this Part of this Act by the Secretary of State has certified in writing that the patient is capable of understanding its nature, purpose and likely effects [*i.e. of the treatment*] and has consented to it; or
(b) a registered medical practitioner appointed as aforesaid (not being the responsible medical officer) has certified in writing that the patient is not capable of understanding the nature, purpose and likely effects of that treatment or has not consented to it but that, having regard to the likelihood of its alleviating or preventing a deterioration of his condition, the treatment should be given.

Section 58(4)
Before giving a certificate under subsection (3)(b) above the registered medical practitioner concerned shall consult two other persons who have been professionally concerned with the patient's medical treatment, and of those persons one shall be a nurse and the other shall be neither a nurse nor a registered medical practitioner.

Section 61
Review of treatment.

Section 61(1)
Where a patient is given treatment in accordance with section 57(2) or 58(3)(b) above a report on the treatment and the patient's condition shall be given by the responsible medical officer to the Secretary of State —
(a) on the next occasion on which the responsible medical officer furnishes a report in respect of the patient under section 20(3) above; and
(b) at any other time if so required by the Secretary of State.

Section 61(2)
[*further details given regarding patients under restriction order or restriction direction*]

Section 62
Urgent treatment [*can be given compulsorily*]

Section 62(1)
Sections 57 and 58 above shall not apply to any treatment —
(a) which is immediately necessary to save the patient's life; or
(b) which (not being irreversible) is immediately necessary to prevent a serious deterioration of his condition; or
(c) which (not being irreversible or hazardous) is immediately necessary to alleviate serious suffering by the patient; or
(d) which (not being irreversible or hazardous) is immediately necessary and represents the minimum interference necessary to prevent the patient from behaving violently or being a danger to himself or to others.

Section 62(3)	For the purposes of this section treatment is irreversible if it has unfavourable irreversible physical or psychological consequences and hazardous if it entails significant physical hazard.
Section 63	**Treatment not requiring consent** The consent of a patient shall not be required for any medical treatment given to him for the mental disorder from which he is suffering, not being treatment falling within section 57 or 58 above, if the treatment is given by or under the direction of the responsible medical officers.

Part V Mental Health Review Tribunals

Section 72

Powers of Tribunals.

Section 72(1)

Where application is made to a Mental Health Review Tribunal by or in respect of a patient who is liable to be detained under this Act, the tribunal may in any case direct that the patient be discharged, and —

(a) the tribunal shall direct the discharge of a patient liable to be detained under section 2 above if they are satisfied —

  (i) that he is not then suffering from mental disorder or from mental disorder of a nature or degree which warrants his detention in a hospital for assessment (or for assessment followed by medical treatment) for at least a limited period; or

  (ii) that his detention as aforesaid is not justified in the interests of his own health or safety or with a view to the protection of other persons;

(b) the tribunal shall direct the discharge of a patient liable to be detained otherwise than under section 2 if they are satisfied —

  (i) that he is not then suffering from mental illness, psychopathic disorder, severe mental impairment or mental impairment or from any of those forms of disorder of a nature or degree which makes it appropriate for him to be liable to be detained in a hospital for medical treatment; or

  (ii) that it is not necessary for the health or safety of the patient or for the protection of other persons that he should receive such treatment; or

  (iii) in the case of an application [*where the RMO (following notice to discharge by the nearest relative) has issued a report certifying that in his opinion the patient, if discharged, would be likely to act in a manner dangerous to other persons or to himself*] that the patient, if released, would not be likely to act in a manner dangerous to other persons or to himself.

Section 72(5)

[*Power to amend an application, order of direction*]

Part VIII Miscellaneous Functions of Local Authorities and the Secretary of State

Section 117

After-care
Refer to the Act and to Appendix I(C). Mental Health (Patients in the Community) Act 1995

Part X Miscellaneous and Supplementary

Section 131

Informal admission of patients.

Section 131(1)

Nothing in this Act shall be construed as preventing a patient who requires treatment for mental disorder from being admitted to any hospital or mental nursing home in pursuance of arrangements made in that behalf and without any application, order or direction rendering him liable to be detained under this Act, or from remaining in any hospital or mental nursing home in pursuance of such arrangements after he has ceased to be so liable to be detained.

Section 135

Warrant to search for and remove patients.

Section 135(6)

[Definition of place of safety]

Section 136

Mentally disordered persons found in public places
[Police powers of arrest. Detention in a place other than hospital.]

Section 139

Protection for acts done in pursuance of this Act

Section 139(1)

No person shall be liable, whether on the ground of want of jurisdiction or on any other ground, to any civil or criminal proceedings to which he would have been liable apart from this section in respect of any act purporting to be done in pursuance of this Act or any regulations or rules made under this Act, or in, or in pursuance or anything done in, the discharge of functions conferred by any other enactment on the authority having jurisdiction under Part VII of this Act, unless the act was done in bad faith or without reasonable care.

Section 139(2)

No civil proceedings shall be brought against any person in any court in respect of any such act without the leave of the High Court; and no criminal proceedings shall be brought against any person in any court in respect of any such act except by or with the consent of the Director of Public Prosecutions.

Section 139(3)

This section does not apply to proceedings for an offence under this Act, being proceedings which, under any other provision of this Act, can be instituted only by or with the consent of the Director of Public Prosecutions.

Section 139(4)

This section does not apply to proceedings against the Secretary of State or against a health authority within the meaning of the National Health Service Act 1977.

Extracts from the Mental Health (Patients in the Community) Act 1995

Section 1(1)　　　　After section 25 of the Mental Health Act 1983 there shall be inserted the following sections —

After-care under supervision

Section 25A(1)　　Where a patient —

(a) is liable to be detained in a hospital in pursuance of an application for admission for treatment; and

(b) has attained the age of 16 years,

an application may be made for him to be supervised after he leaves hospital, for the period allowed by the following provisions of this Act, with a view to securing that he receives the after-care services provided to him under section 117 below.

Section 25A(2)　　In this Act an application for a patient to be so supervised is referred to as a "supervision application"; and where a supervision application has been duly made and accepted under this Part of this Act in respect of a patient and he has left hospital, he is for the purposes of this Act "subject to after-care under supervision" (until he ceases to be so subject in accordance with the provisions of this Act).

Section 25A(3)　　A supervision application shall be made in accordance with this section and sections 25B and 25C below.

Section 25A(4)　　A supervision application may be made in respect of a patient only on the grounds that —

(a) he is suffering from mental disorder, being mental illness, severe mental impairment, psychopathic disorder or mental impairment;

(b) there would be substantial risk of serious harm to the health or safety of the patient or the safety or other persons, or of the patient being seriously exploited, if he were not to receive the after-care services to be provided for him under section 117 below after he leaves hospital; and

(c) his being subject to after-care under supervision is likely to help to secure that he receives the after-care services to be so provided.

Section 25A(5)　　A supervision application may be made only by the responsible medical officer.

Section 25A(6)	A supervision application in respect of a patient shall be addressed to the Health Authority which will have the duty under section 117 below to provide after-care services for the patient after he leaves hospital.
Section 25A(7)	Before accepting a supervision application in respect of a patient a Health Authority shall consult the local social services authority which will also have that duty.
Section 25A(8)	Where a Health Authority accepts a supervision application in respect of a patient the Health Authority shall —

(a) inform the patient both orally and in writing —

    (i) that the supervision application has been accepted; and

    (ii) of the effect in his case of the provisions of this Act relating to a patient subject to after-care under supervision (including, in particular, what rights of applying to a Mental Health Review Tribunal are available);

(b) inform any person whose name is stated in the supervision application in accordance with sub-paragraph (i) of paragraph (e) of section 25B(5) below that the supervision application has been accepted; and

(c) inform in writing any person whose name is so stated in accordance with sub-paragraph (ii) of that paragraph that the supervision application has been accepted.

Section 25A(9)	*Provision for Section 17 patients.*

Making of supervision application

Section 25B(1)	The responsible medical officer shall not make a supervision application unless —

(a) subsection (2) below is complied with; and

(b) the responsible medical officer has considered the matters specified in subsection (4) below.

Section 25B(2)	This subsection is complied with if —

(a) the following persons have been consulted about the making of the supervision application —

    (i) the patient;

    (ii) one or more persons who have been professionally concerned with the patient's medical treatment in hospital;

    (iii) one or more persons who will be professionally concerned with the after-care services to be provided for the patient under section 117 below; and

    (iv) any person who the responsible medical officer believes will play a substantial part in the care of the patient after he leaves hospital but will not be professionally concerned with any of the after-care services to be so provided;

(b)   such steps as are practicable have been taken to consult the person (if any) appearing to be the nearest relative of the patient about the making of the supervision application; and

(c)   the responsible medical officer has taken into account any views expressed by the persons consulted.

Section 25B(3)   Where the patient has requested that paragraph (b) of subsection (2) above should not apply, that paragraph shall not apply unless —

(a)   the patient has a propensity to violent or dangerous behaviour towards others; and

(b)   the responsible medical officer considers that it is appropriate for steps such as are mentioned in that paragraph to be taken.

Section 25B(4)   The matters referred to in subsection (1)(b) above are —

(a)   the after-care services to be provided for the patient under section 117 below; and

(b)   any requirements to be imposed on him under section 25D below.

Section 25B(5)   A supervision application shall state —

(a)   that the patient is liable to be detained in a hospital in pursuance of an application for admission for treatment;

(b)   the age of the patient, or, if his exact age is not known to the applicant, that the patient is believed to have attained the age of 16 years;

(c)   that in the opinion of the applicant (having regard in particular to the patient's history) all of the conditions set out in section 25A(4) above are complied with;

(d)   the name of the person who is to be community responsible medical officer, and of the person who is to be the supervisor, in relation to the person after he leaves hospital; and

(e)   the name of —

(i)   any person who has been consulted under paragraph (a)(iv) of subsection (2) above; and

(ii)   any person who has been consulted under paragraph (b) of that subsection.

Section 25B(6)   A supervision application shall be accompanied by —

(a)   the written recommendation in the prescribed form of a registered medical practitioner who will be professionally concerned with the patient's medical treatment after he leaves hospital or, if no such practitioner other than the responsible medical officer will be so concerned, of any registered medical practitioner, and

(b)   the written recommendation in the prescribed form of an approved social worker.

Section 25B(7)   A recommendation under subsection (6)(a) above shall include a statement that in the opinion of the medical practitioner (having regard in particular to the patient's history) all the conditions set out in section 25A(4) above are complied with.

Section 25B(8)   A recommendation under subsection (6)(b) above shall include a statement that in the opinion of the social worker (having regard in particular to the patient's history) both of the conditions set out in section 25A(4)(b) and (c) above are complied with.

Section 25B(9)   A supervision application shall also be accompanied by —

(a) a statement in writing by the person who is to be the community responsible medical officer in relation to the patient after he leaves hospital that he is to be in charge of the medical treatment provided for the patient as part of the after-care services provided for him under section 117 below;

(b) a statement in writing to the person who is to be the supervisor in relation to the patient after he leaves hospital that he is to supervise the patient with a view to securing that he receives the after-care services so provided;

(c) details of the after-care services to be provided for the patient under section 117 below; and

(d) details of any requirement to be imposed on him under section 25D below.

Section 25B(10)   On making a supervision application in respect of a patient the responsible medical officer shall —

(a) inform the patient both orally and in writing;

(b) inform any person who has been consulted under paragraph (a)(iv) of subsection (2) above; and

(c) inform in writing any person who has been consulted under paragraph (b) of that subsection,

of the matters specified in subsection (11) below.

Section 25B(11)   The matters specified in subsection (10) above are —

(a) that the application is being made;

(b) the after-care service to be provided for the patient under section 117 below;

(c) any requirements to be imposed on him under section 25D below; and

(d) the name of the person who is to be the community responsible medical officer, and of the person who is to be the supervisor, in relation to the patient after he leaves hospital.

Supervision applications: supplementary

Section 25C   *Covers supplementary provisions on the supervision application, relating to the form of mental disorder, the right of the doctor or approved social worker to visit the patient at any reasonable time, and provision for rectification of the supervision application within 14 days.*

Requirements to secure receipt of after-care under supervision

Section 25D   *This section gives powers to those bodies providing* after-care to impose the requirements specified, ie. the patient resides at a specified place, attends a specified place for medical treatment, occupational therapy, education or training. Access can be given to any registered medical practitioner, approved social worker or other person authorized by the supervisor. Powers are given to take the patient to and from the place specified for treatment, etc.

Section 25E	**Review of after-care under supervision etc** *Duty on the responsible after-care bodies to keep the patient under review.*
Section 25F	**Reclassification of patient subject to after-care under supervision** *Provides for the reclassification of a patient subject to after-care under supervision if the form of mental disorder is different from that specified.*
Section 25G	**Duration and renewal of after-care under supervision** *Duration and renewal of after-care under supervision, beginning when he leaves hospital and ending with the period of six months beginning with the day on which the supervision application was accepted. Supervision can be renewed for a further six months and then for a year at a time if specified conditions are present.*
Section 25H	**Ending of after-care under supervision** *Community responsible medical officer can end the after-care supervision at any time.*
Section 25I	**Special provisions as to patients sentenced to imprisonment etc** A patient detained in prison after imprisonment or remand or a patient detained in hospital after an application for admission for assessment (section 2) who are already subject to after-care under supervision, is not required to receive section 117 services or after-care under supervision.
Section 25J	**Patients moving from Scotland to England and Wales** – a supervision application can be made if they are subject to a community care order in Scotland.
Section 2	**Absence without leave** *This amends Section 18 of the 1983 Act to allow a patient to be taken into custody at any time up to six months from the date he absconded.*
Section 3	**Leave of absence from hospital** *This amends section 17 to remove the limit of six months on the period for which leave of absence may be granted.*
Section 4, 5 and 6	Scotland.
Section 7	Act comes into force 1 April 1996.
Schedules	1 After-care under supervision: supplementary provisions. 2 Community care orders (Scotland): supplementary provisions.

Paragraph	Nature of duty	Responsible body
	A. Assessment	
Para 2.11	Guidance to approved social workers (ASWs) on where assistance from professional interpreter can be obtained	Local Authority
Para 2.14	Displacing nearest relative	Local Authority County Court
Para 2.33a	Request for nearest relative under section 13(4)	Local Authority
Para 2.33b	Response to repeated requests for assessment	Local Authority
Para 2.33c	Acceptance of requests from nearest relatives via GPs or other professionals	Local Authority
Para 2.35	Guidance on use of interpreters	Local Authority
Para 2.40	Records to be kept of ethnicity of patients	NHS Trusts Local Authority
	B. Part III Assessments	
Para 3.4	Up-to-date information on facilities available	Regional Authority Welsh Office
	C. Police powers of arrest – Section 136	
Para 10.1	Implementation of section 136	LA/DHA/Police
Para 10.19	Invoking power of section 135	Local Authority
	D. Conveying to hospital	
Para 11.3	Joint policy/procedure on conveying to hospital covering roles and obligations	LA/DHA
	E. Receipt and scrutiny of documents	
Para 12.1	Delegation of duties to receive and scrutinize documents	Managers/DHA
	F. Guardianship	
Para 13.6	Arrangements for receiving, considering and scrutinizing applications, for monitoring etc.	Local Authority
	G. Treatment and care in hospital	
Para 14.3	System to ensure implementation of statutory responsibilities to inform	Hospital managers

Para 16.19	Devise form to cover treatment in an emergency under section 62	Hospital managers
Para 16.33b	Devise system to remind RMO prior to expiry of limits set by section 58 and 61	Hospital managers
Para 16.33c	Devise system to remind *re* patient consent or second opinion required	Hospital managers
Para 18.13	Clear written policies on use of restraint	Hospital managers
Para 18.16	Clear written guidelines on use of seclusion	Hospital managers
Para 18.29b	Written guidelines distinguishing categories for physically secure conditions	Hospital managers
Para 18.33	Clear written operational policy on all forms of restraint	Hospital managers
Para 19.2	Guidelines for procedures to note and monitor use of behaviour modification programmes	Hospital managers
Para 19.10	Clear written policies on use of time-out as part of their overall policy on general management	Hospital managers

H. Absence without leave – section 18

Para 21.2	Clear written policy in relation to action to be taken when a detained patient goes absent without leave	Hospital managers/LA

I. Managers' duty to review detention

Para 22.5	How to review	Hospital managers

J. Correspondence

Para 24.15	Written policy on implementation of power to withhold mail	Hospital managers

K. Personal searches

Para 25.1	Operational policy on searching of patients and their belongings	Hospital managers

L. Visiting patients

Para 26.5	Managers' duty to monitor exclusion of visitors	Hospital managers

M. After-care

Para 27.3	Agreed procedures for establishing after-care arrangements	HA/NHS Trusts and Social Services Authority

Note: LA – Local Authority
DHA – District Health Authority

<table>
<tr><td>

**Appendix
I(D)**

</td><td>

Law Commission Report No. 231, Mental Incapacity 1995 HMSO

</td></tr>
</table>

<table>
<tr><td>

Contents

</td><td>

Part I   Introduction – scope, history & structure of the report
Part II   Content and basic approach to reform
Part III   Two fundamental concepts:
- Lack of capacity
- Best interests

Part IV   General authority to act reasonably
Part V   Advance statements about healthcare (i.e. 'Living Wills')
Part VI   Independent supervision of medical and research procedure
Part VII   Continuing Power of Attorney
Part VIII   Decision making by the Court
Part IX   Public protection for vulnerable people at risk
Part X   The Judicial Forum
Part XI   Collected recommendations

</td></tr>
<tr><td>

**Appendix A
Draft Mental
Incapacity Bill**

</td><td>

The draft Mental Incapacity Bill contained in Appendix A of the Law Commission's Report No 231 covers the following clauses:

Part I   Mental Incapacity – definition and action to be taken in best interests of such persons
General authority to provide care but restriction on this general authority
Non-therapeutic procedures
Continuing power of attorney
General power of the courts and appointment of manager
Miscellaneous and supplementary provisions

Part II   Persons in need of care and attention

Part III   Jurisdiction of magistrates' court and Court of Protection

Part IV   General interpretation and treatment provisions
Eight schedules

</td></tr>
<tr><td>

Comment

</td><td>

Implementation of these provisions would fill the vacuum which currently exists in relation to the decision making on behalf of an adult with mental incapacity. The Law Commission expressed the hope that the Bill might be implemented in January 1996 but this will obviously not come to pass.

</td></tr>
</table>

Appendix II Forms and leaflets with examples of non-statutory forms

Chapter 4	**Admission to hospital under Part II of the Act**
Statutory Form No.	*Description*

	Application for admission for assessment MHA 1983 Section 2 and 4: Set of Pink forms
1	By nearest relative
2	By approved social worker
3	Joint medical recommendation
4	Medical recommendation
5	Emergency application by nearest relative
6	Emergency application by approved social worker
7	Medical recommendation/emergency admission for assessment

	Application for admission for treatment MHA 1983 Section 3: Set of Pink forms
8	By nearest relative
9	By approved social worker
10	Joint medical recommendation
11	Medical recommendation
12	Application for formal admission of in-patient (section 5(2)
13	Emergency application for formal admission of in-patient (section 5(4))
14	Record of admission (section 2, 3, 4 and 5(2))
15	Record of receipt of medical recommendations (sections 2, 3, 4 and 7)
16	Record of time at which power to detain under MHA 1983 section 5(4) elapsed
22	Reclassification of patient detained for treatment (section 16)
30	Renewal of authority for detention (section 20)

176

Chapter 6	**Provision of information to the patient and nearest relative**
Example	*Description*
A	Leaflet for conveying information to detained patients MHA 1983 Leaflet 1, section 5(4)
B	Form recording information given and patient's understanding **including** record of patient's request that nearest relative is **not** informed of detention and/or discharge Example from Powys Health Care NHS Trust 'Patients Rights – Proforma for Informing'
C	Form recording compulsory treatment under section 62 Example from Powys Health Care NHS Trust 'Section 62: Urgent Treatment of Mental Disorder'

Chapter 8	**Consent to treatment**
Statutory Form No.	*Description*
38	Form recording patient's consent to treatment under section 58, MHA 1983 Section 58(3)(a)
39	Form recording second opinion doctor's authority for treatment in the absence of patient's consent under section 58, MHA 1983 section 58(3)(b)
MHAC 1	Mental Health Act Commission Form 1: Mental Health Act 1983 Review of treatment (section 61)

Chapter 9	**Appeals against detention**
Statutory Form No.	*Description*
MHRT 1	MHRT Application Form 1: Patients detained under section 2
MHRT 2	MHRT Application Form 2: Patients detained under section 3, 37, 47 or 48
Example	*Description*
D	Example from Powys Health Care NHS Trust
E	Example from Powys Health Care NHS Trust

Chapter 10   **Leave with consent under section 17**

Example	*Description*
F	Form for recording section 17 leave Example from Powys Health Care NHS Trust

Chapter 13   **Police powers of arrest**

Example	*Description*
G	Application for admission to place of safety (use of section 136) Example from Powys Health Care NHS Trust

Chapter 14   **Transfer of patients**

Statutory Form No.	*Description*
24	Transfer Hospital to Hospital, Form 24 Parts I and II, MHA 1983 section 19
25	Transfer Hospital to Guardianship, Form 25 Parts I–III, MHA 1983 section 19
26	Transfer Guardianship to Guardianship, Form 26 Parts I–III, MHA 1983 section 19
27	Transfer Guardianship to Hospital, Form 27, MHA 1983 Section 19

Chapter 17   **Community care**

Example	*Description*
H	A typical form for implementing section 117 (After-care), abridged – full form is 13 pages

Chapter 20   **The Mental Health Act Commission**

Example	*Description*
J	Mental Health Act Commission Visit announcement Example from Powys Health Care NHS Trust

Example A: MHA 1983 Leaflet 1

Mental Health Act 1983 Leaflet 1
Section 5(4)

Name ....

Your hospital doctor is ....

His nominated deputy is ....

Date .... Time when holding power started ....

Your rights under
the Mental Health Act 1983

Why you are being held

You are being held in this hospital/mental nursing home for up to six hours so that you can be seen by a doctor. You must not leave during this time unless a doctor or nurse tells you that you can. If you try to leave before then the staff can stop you, and if you do leave you can be brought back. You can be held in this way because of Section 5(4) of the Mental Health Act 1983. These notes are to tell you what that means.

If the doctor does not see you within these six hours you will be free to go, but if you want to go, please talk to a nurse first. When the doctor sees you he may say that you need to stay in hospital for a longer time. If he does, he will tell you why, and for how long it is likely to be, and you will be given a further leaflet to explain your rights. If he decides you do not need to stay he will talk to you about what other help you should have.

If you have any questions or complaints

If you want to ask something, or to complain about something, talk to the doctor, nurse or social worker. If you are not happy with the answer you may write to the hospital managers. You may do this even after the six hours is over.
Their address is

....

....

If you are still not happy with the reply you are given you can ask the Mental Health Act Commission to help you. You can also write to the Commission even after you have left hospital.

The Mental Health Act Commission
The Commission was set up specially to make sure that the mental health law is used properly and that patients are cared for properly while they are kept in hospital. You can ask them to help you by writing to them at

. . . .

. . . .

. . . .

Your nearest relative
A copy of these notes will be sent to your nearest relative who we have been told is

. . . .

If you do not want this to happen please tell the nurse in charge of your ward or a doctor.

If there is anything in this leaflet you do not understand, the doctor or a nurse or social worker will help you. If you need help in writing a letter you should ask one of them, or a relative or friend.

Example B

PATIENTS RIGHTS – PROFORMA FOR INFORMING
MENTAL HEALTH ACT 1983

.... who is detained under

Section .... has been issued with leaflet number(s) .... at .... am/pm

on (date) .... and his/her rights under the Mental Health

Act 1983 have been explained to him/her.

*(1)   He/She appears to have understood this explanation/
*(2)   He/She has refused to accept this explanation/
*(3)   He/She does not appear to have understood this explanation.

Action on (2) or (3) above: Further attempts made on:

Date: ....   Time: ....

Date: ....   Time: ....

*(1)   He/She appears to have understood this explanation/
*(2)   He/She has refused to accept this explanation/
*(3)   He/She does not appear to have understood this explanation.

NB: When the patient has accepted this explanation please indicate whether or not the patient's relative is to be informed.

*Yes/No – Name of relative to be informed: ....

Signed: ....   Designation: ....
                                     (First Level Nurse)
Signed: ....   (Patient)

Signed: ....   (Administrator)

A note of the above must be placed in the patient's nursing notes.

* Please delete as appropriate.

Example C

MENTAL HEALTH ACT 1983

SECTION 62
URGENT TREATMENT OF MENTAL DISORDER

Name of patient: .... Ward: ....

Date of detention: .... Section: ....

Patients RMO: ....

Doctor Prescribing Treatment: ....

Reason for giving treatment: ....

....

....

....

....

....

Prescribed treatment: ....

....

....

Was the RMO consulted beforehand?   Yes/No

Has a Second Opinion Appointed Doctor (SOAD) been requested   Yes/No

Signature: ....

Designation: .... Date: ....

This form should be sent to the Hospital Managers, and a copy placed in the case-notes.

Reproduced with permission from Powys Health Care NHS Trust.

Example D: MHRT 1

Application for Mental Health Review Tribunal from patient detained under section 2 of the Mental Health Act 1983

Application Form

Please complete this form as far as you are able. If you are unsure how to complete it you can ask anyone at the hospital, a relative or a friend for help.

1. I am being detained in hospital under section 2 of the Mental Health Act 1983 and I wish to apply for a Mental Health Review Tribunal.

2. My full name is ....

3. The name and address of the hospital or mental nursing home in which I am detained is

....

....

....

....

4. The detention began on .... (give date)

5. My nearest relative is my .... and his/her
                                              (state relationship)
    name and address is

....

....

....

....

If your nearest relative, or if a court, has appointed someone else to act as a nearest relative, please put his or her name and address.

6. **If you would like to appoint someone, for example a solicitor, to represent you at the Tribunal hearing, the Tribunal Office or a social worker can tell you how to find one. Because of the legal advice and assistance scheme the solicitor's help may be free or it may only cost you a little.**

If you have appointed someone to represent you at the Tribunal hearing please give his/her name and address

. . . .

. . . .

. . . .

. . . .

If you do not have anyone to represent you please tick one of the following boxes

i. I am going to appoint someone to represent me at the Tribunal hearing (please send the name and address of the representative to the Tribunal Office as soon as possible)

or

ii. I do not wish to be represented

Signed . . . .

Date . . . .

When completed this form should be sent to: **Mental Health Review Tribunal**

Example E: MHRT 2

Application for Mental Health Review Tribunal from patient detained in hospital for treatment under section 3, 37, 47 or 48 of the Mental Health Act 1983, or treated as if detained under one of those sections.

Application Form

Please complete this form as far as you are able. If you are unsure how to complete it you can ask anyone at the hospital, a relative or a friend for help.

1. I am detained in a hospital or a mental nursing home for treatment under the Mental Health Act 1983 and I wish to apply for a Mental Health Review Tribunal.

2. My full name is . . . .

3. The name and address of the hospital or mental nursing home in which I am detained is

. . . .

. . . .

. . . .

. . . .

4. I am detained under section . . . . of the Mental Health Act 1983 (if known)

5. My nearest relative is my . . . . and his/her name and address is
    (state relationship)

. . . .

. . . .

. . . .

. . . .

If your nearest relative, or if a court, has appointed someone else to act as a nearest relative, please put his or her name and address.

6. **If you would like to appoint someone, for example a solicitor, to represent you at the Tribunal hearing, the Tribunal Office or a social worker can tell you how to find one. Because of the legal advice and assistance scheme the solicitor's help may be free or it may only cost you a little.**

If you have appointed someone to represent you at the Tribunal hearing, please give his/her name and address

. . . .

. . . .

. . . .

. . . .

If you do not have anyone to represent you please tick one of the following boxes

i.   I am going to appoint someone to represent me at the Tribunal hearing (please send the name and address of the representative to the Tribunal Office as soon as possible)

or

ii.   I do not wish to be represented

Signed . . . .

Date . . . .

When completed this form should be sent to: **Mental Health Review Tribunal**

Example F: Form for recording section 17 leave

**POWYS HEALTH CARE NHS TRUST
MID WALES HOSPITAL**

TO THE MANAGERS

Order for the Leave of Absence of a patient on Section, in compliance with Section 17 of the Mental Health Act 1983.

Name of Patient: . . . .

Detained under Section . . . . of the Mental Health Act 1983.

I, being the Consultant in Charge, hereby authorise leave of absence in respect of the above-named as follows:

Details of dates of authorised leave:

. . . .

. . . .

. . . .

Signed: . . . . Consultant in Charge

Date: . . . .

- -

Recorded in patients notes – date: . . . .

Sent to Locality Administrator – date: . . . .

Signed: . . . .
Sister/Charge Nurse/Staff Nurse

- -

For Office Use:

Copy returned to ward for casenotes

Signed: . . . .   Date: . . . .

Example G: Application for admission to a place of safety

MENTAL HEALTH ACT 1983

APPLICATION FOR ADMISSION TO A PLACE OF SAFETY
SECTION 136

To: The Managers of Mid Wales Hospital, Talgarth

I, Police . . . . of the Dyfed-Powys Constabulary,

hereby apply for the admission of . . . .

of . . . .

to Mid Wales Hospital in accordance with the provisions of Section 136 of the Mental Health Act 1983.

Signed: . . . .

Date: . . . . Time: . . . .

- -

RECORD OF ADMISSION
SECTION 136

. . . . was

admitted to Mid Wales Hospital, Talgarth, in pursuance of this application at . . . . am/pm

on . . . .

Signed: . . . . (On behalf of the Managers)

Date: . . . .

Consultant notified:	Date:	Time: . . . .
Senior Nurse notified:	Date:	Time: . . . .
ASW notified:	Date:	Time: . . . .

Example H: Implementing section 117 after-care

POWYS HEALTH CARE NHS TRUST/POWYS SOCIAL SERVICES DEPARTMENT

MENTAL HEALTH ACT 1983

SECTION 117 – JOINT AFTERCARE PROCEDURE

**APPENDIX 1: NOTIFICATION OF ENTITLEMENT TO AFTERCARE
UNDER SECTION 117**

To: Nurse in Charge (Patient's File)

Patient's Name: ....

Section: ....

Date of Section: ....

Hospital Number: ....

Ward: ....

The above-named is subject to Aftercare under Section 117 of the Mental Health Act 1983. Your attention is drawn to the Joint Procedure which gives details of the action required.

.... Date: ....
        Locality Administrator

Copies to:

Responsible Medical Officer
Area Care Manager (who will inform Director of Social Services)
Appropriate Community Mental Health Team Leader

APPENDIX 2: INDIVIDUAL INFORMATION AND DISCHARGE PLAN

Copies to (please tick as appropriate):

Responsible Medical Officer (name) ....

Key Worker (please specify

CPN/Social Worker and name) ....

GP (name) ....

Patient's Medical Records File

---

1   **NAME** .... DoB ....

ADDRESS ....

....

NEAREST RELATIVE/REPRESENTATIVE ....

ADDRESS ....

....

ADMISSION DATE .... SECTION .... WARD ....

---

2   **MDT MEMBERS** [*multi-disciplinary team*]

CONSULTANT .... PRIMARY WORKER ....

SOCIAL WORKER .... CPN ....

DESIGNATED COMMUNITY KEY WORKER ....

OTHERS ....

....

....

Summary of further headings in Appendix 2

3   **PRIMARY CASE CONFERENCE**
(date, those present, summary, name community key worker, date notification received)

4   **INTERIM CASE CONFERENCE**
(date, those present, summary)

5 **PRE-DISCHARGE (FINAL CASE CONFERENCE)**
(date, those present, after-care requirements that will be provided, aftercare requirements needed but not available)
Signatures – Primary Nurse and Community Key Worker
Summary
Notification to other Health Authority/Trust and Social Services (where applicable)

6 **POST-DISCHARGE CASE CONFERENCE**
(date, those present)
(a) Review of progress from discharge
(b) Work undertaken/employment
(c) Goals achieved
(d) Community involvements e.g. day attendance
(e) Future objective agreed with client
Signatures RMO/Community Key Worker

APPENDIX 3: INDIVIDUAL INFORMATION AND DISCHARGE PLAN – CHECKLIST

	YES	NO	PERSON RESPONSIBLE	COMMENTS	DATE
1 MDT Meetings Primary Interim Final (pre-discharge) Post Discharge					
2 Trial Leave					
3 Is assistance with any of the following required? Accommodation Employment Finance Family Circumstances					
4 Community Support – Are any of the following supports involved and/or needed? Relatives/Carer/Friends CPN Social Worker Psychiatrist Paramedics Occupational Therapist Day Hospital Other					
5 Medication Requirements Will the client need medication on discharge? Has the client's GP been notified?					

Headings of remaining sections

Appendix 4: Record of Refusal of After-care
Appendix 5: Report by Key Worker following 6 months discharge from hospital
Appendix 6: Notice of discharge from section 117
Appendix 7: Notification case conference (Medical Secretary)
Appendix 8: Notification case conference (Individual)

[*The Powys Health Care NHS Trust Form is 13 pages in length*]

Example J: MHAC visit announcement
As sent to all detained patients prior to MHAC's visits

Date:

Dear

Re: <u>Mental Health Act Commissioners Visit – September 199–</u>

The Mental Health Act Commissioners are making their annual visit to the hospital in September 199–.

They will be available for private interview should you wish to see them, or should you wish any items to be brought to their attention please contact Mrs xxxxxx, Locality Administrator.

Please complete the bottom portion of this letter, and return it in the enclosed addressed envelope as soon as possible.

Yours sincerely

xxxxxx (Mrs)
Locality Administrator

- -

<u>Mental Health Act Commissioners Visit – September 199–</u>

*I do/do not wish any items to be brought to the attention of the Mental Health Act Commissioners.

*I do/do not wish to have an interview with the Mental Health Act Commissioners.

Signed: . . . .

* Please delete as applicable

Useful Addresses

Alzheimer's Disease Society
Gordon House,
10 Greencoat Place,
London SW1P 1PH
Tel. 0171-306 0606

Association of Directors of Social Services,
Social Services Dept.,
North Yorkshire County Council,
County Hall,
Northallerton,
N. Yorks DL7 8DD
Tel. (01609) 770661
Fax (01609) 773158

Association of Mental Health Act Administrators
c/o Mental Health Act Administrator,
The Maudsley Hospital,
Denmark Hill,
London SE5 8AZ

British Association of Social Workers
16 Kent Street,
Birmingham B5 6RD
Tel. 0121-622 3911
Fax 0121 622 4860

British Institute of Learning Disabilities (BILD)
Wolverhampton Road,
Kidderminster,
Worcs. DY10 3PP
Tel. (01562) 850251
Fax (01562) 951970

Counsel and Care for the Elderly
Twyman House,
16 Bonny Street,
London NW1 9PG
Tel. 0171-485 1550

English National Board
Victory House,
170 Tottenham Court Road,
London W1P 0HA
Tel. 0171-388 3131
Fax 0171-383 4031

Good Practices in Mental Health
380–384 Harrow Road,
London W9 2HU
Tel. 0171-289 2034/3060

Headway (National Head Injuries Association)
7 King Edward Court,
King Edward Street,
Nottingham NG1 1EW
Tel. 0115-924 0800

Health Service Commissioner (the Ombudsman) (England)
Church House,
Great Smith Street, London SW1P 3BW
Tel. 0171-276 2035

Health Service Commissioner (the Ombudsman) (Wales)
4th Floor,
Pearl Assurance House,
Grey Friars Road,
Cardiff CF1 3AG

MENCAP (see Royal Society of Mentally Handicapped Children and Adults)

Mental After Care Association
25 Bedford Street,
London WC1B 3HW
Tel. 0171-436 6194

Mental Health Act Commission
Maid Marian House,
56 Hounds Gate,
Nottingham NG1 6BG
Tel. 0115-950 4040
Fax 0115-950 5998

Mental Health Foundation
37 Mortimer Street, London W1N 7RJ
Tel. 0171-580 0145
Fax 0171-631 3868

Mental Health Review Tribunals

Liverpool
3rd Floor,
Cressington House,
249 St. Mary's Road,
Garston,
Liverpool L19 0NF
Tel. 0151-494 0095

London (North)
Spur 3,
Block I,
Government Buildings,
Honeypot Lane,
Stanmore,
Middlesex HA7 1AY
Tel. 0171-972 3738

London (South)
Block 3,
Crown Offices,
Kingston Bypass Road,
Surbiton,
Surrey KT6 5QN
Tel. 0181-398 4166

Nottingham
Spur A,
Block 5,
Government Buildings,
Chalfont Drive,
Western Boulevard,
Nottingham NG8 3RZ
Tel. 0115-929 4222

Wales
1st Floor,
New Crown Buildings,
Cathays Park,
Cardiff CF1 3NQ
Tel. (01222) 823036

MIND National Association for Mental Health
Granta House,
15–19 Broadway,
Stratford,
London E15 4BQ
Tel. 0181-519 2122

National Association of Crossroads Caring for Carers
10 Regents Place,
Rugby
Tel (01778) 573653

National Association for Voluntary Hostels
Fulham Palace,
Bishops Avenue,
London SW6 6EA
Tel. 071-731 4205

National Autistic Society
276 Willesden Lane,
London NW2 5RB
Tel. 0181-451 1114

National Council for Voluntary Organisations
Regents Wharf,
8 All Saints Street,
London N1 9RL
Tel. 0171-713 6161

National Schizophrenia Fellowship
28 Castle Street,
Kingston upon Thames,
Surrey KT1 1SS
Tel. 0181-547 3973
Fax 0181-574 3862

Ombudsman (See Health Service Commissioner)

Registered Nursing Homes
Calthorpe House,
Hagley Road,
Edgbaston,
Birmingham B16 8QY
Tel. 0121-454 2511
Fax 0121-454 0932

Richmond Fellowship for Community Mental Health
8 Addison Road,
London W14 8DL
Tel. 0171-603 6373
Fax 0171-602 8652

Royal Society for Mentally Handicapped Children and Adults (MENCAP)
National Centre,
123 Golden Lane,
London EC1Y 0RT
Tel. 0171-454 0454
Fax 071-3254

United Kingdom Central Council for Nursing, Midwifery and Health Visiting
23 Portland Place,
London W1N 3AF
Tel. 0171-637 7181
Fax 0171-436 2924

English National Board for Nursing, Midwifery and Health Visiting
Victory House,
170 Tottenham Court Road,
London W1P 0HA
Tel. 0171-388 3131

Welsh National Board for Nursing, Midwifery and Health Visiting
Floor 13,
Pearl Assurance House,
Greyfriars Road,
Cardiff CF1 3AG
Tel. (01222) 395535
Fax (01222) 229366

Scottish National Board for Nursing, Midwifery and Health Visiting
22 Queen Street,
Edinburgh EH2 1NT
Tel. 0131-226 7371

National Board for Nursing, Midwifery and Health Visiting for Northern Ireland
79 Chichester Street,
Belfast BT1 4JE
Tel. (01232) 238152

Bibliography

Audit Commission (1994) *Finding a Place: a review of the Mental Health Service for Adults*, London, HMSO.

Blom-Cooper L. (1992) *Report of Inquiry into Ashworth Hospital*, London, HMSO.

Blom-Cooper, L. (1995) *Falling Shadow, Inquiry of Events at Edith Morgan Unit, Torbay.* HMSO.

Bluglass, R. (1992) *A Guide to the Mental Health Act*, Edinburgh, Churchill Livingstone.

Brazier, M. (1992) *Medicine, Patients and the Law*, Middlesex, Penguin Books.

Department of Health (1989) *Caring for People*, London, HMSO.

Department of Health (1993) *Code of Practice on the Mental Health Act 1983*, 2nd edn., Department of Health and Welsh Office.

Department of Health (1994) *Being Heard* (report of the Wilson Committee), HMSO.

Department of Health (1995) *Statistical Bulletin: In-patients Formally Detained in Hospital Under the Mental Health Act 1983 and Other Legislation, England 1987–88 to 1992–93*, London, HMSO.

DHSS Memorandum (1983) *The Mental Health Act*, London, HMSO.

Dimond, B.C. (1995) *Legal Aspects of Nursing*, 2nd edn., Hemel Hempstead, Prentice Hall.

Dimond, B.C. (1993) *Patients' Rights, Responsibilities and the Nurse*, Lancaster, Central Health Studies series, Quay Publishing.

Gann, R. (1993) *The NHS A to Z*, 2nd edn., The Help for Health Trust.

Gostin, L., Rassaby, E. and Buchan, A. *A Mental Health Tribunal Procedure*, Oyez Longman Practice Notes, Harlow, Longman.

Ham, C. (1991) *The New National Health Service*, National Association of Health Authority Trusts (NAHAT).

Hoggett, B. (1994) *Mental Health Law*, London, Sweet & Maxwell.

Hunt, G. & Wainwright, P. (eds.) (1994) *Expanding the Role of the Nurse*, Oxford, Blackwell Science.

Jones, R. (1994) *Mental Health Act Manual*, 4th edn., London, Sweet & Maxwell.

Law Commission *Reports on the Incapacitated Adult: Decision Making* No. 119 (1991), No. 128, No. 129, and No. 130 (1993), London, HMSO.

Law Commission *Report on Mental Incapacity* No. 231 (1995), London, HMSO.

Mental Health Act (1983) London, HMSO.

Pyne, R.H. (1991) *Professional Discipline in Nursing, Midwifery and Health Visiting*, 2nd edn., Oxford, Blackwell Science.

Ritchie, J., Dick, D. and Lingham, R. (1994) *The Report of the Inquiry into the Care and Treatment of Christopher Clunis*, London, HMSO.

Rowson, R. (1990) *An Introduction to Ethics for Nurses*, Harrow, Scutari Press.

Rumbold, G. (1993) *Ethics in Nursing Practice*, 2nd ed., London, Baillière Tindall.

Select Committee of House of Lords (1994) *Medical Ethics: Report of Session 1993/94*, London, HMSO.

Mental Health Review Tribunal Rules 1983 (SI 1983 No. 942), London, HMSO.

Williamson, C. (1991) *Hearing Patients' Appeals against continued compulsory detention*, 2nd edn., National Association of Health Authority Trusts (NAHAT).

Young, A.P. (1994) *Law and Professional Conduct in Nursing*, 2nd edn., Harrow, Scutari Press.

Reference should also be made to publications from MIND (see Useful Addresses).

Index

Entries in bold indicate main references to a topic.

Absence without leave, **86–91**

Acts (*see* Table of Statutes)

Admission, 2, 3, 6, 9, **14–24**, 29, 30–31, 79
application by approved social worker, 110–111
application by nearest relative for, 54
checklists, **124–7**
forms, 121–3, 176
mentally disordered offenders, 33–44
records, 79, 100–102

Aftercare, 4, 9, 50, 57, 117–18, 120
form for section 117, 116, 189–92

Appeals, 45, 54, 56, **72–81**, 129, 131
against tribunal decision, 78

Approved doctor (*see* SOAD)

Approved social worker, 49, 54, 87, 92–3, 102, **110–114**

Arrest, 89, **95–99**

Ashworth enquiry, 33, 136

Assessment
admission for, 9, 20, 22, **24–26**, 54
checklist, admission for, 124–5
of need, 115

ASW (*see* approved social worker)

Audit Commission, 119

Bolam test, 48, 150, 152

Care (*see* after-care, community, multidisciplinary, social services)

Case conference, 116, 190, 191

Cases (*see* Table of Cases), 116, 190, 191

Children (*see* minors)

Clozepine, 9, 62

Code of Practice, 1, **6–9**, **20**, **23**, **27**, **28**, **30**, **45**, **60**, **66**, **70**, 80, **84**, **85**, **116**, **129**, 133, 134, 173–4

Commission (*see* Mental Health Act Commission)

Community care, 4, 18, 30, 82, 90, 110–113, **115–120**, 130, 134, 148, 178
supervision orders, 36, 117–118

Complaints, 9, 45, **48**, 130, 131, **134–7**

Consent
leave with, **82–5**
leave without, **86–91**

Consent to treatment, 3, 21, 25, 26, **59–71**, 113, 118, 134
checklists, 130, 131
forms, 64–5, 177
information about, 45, 46, 48

Consent to transfer, 102–3

Definitions
assault and battery, 59
insanity, 35
managers, 79, 129
mental disorder, 2, 12, **13–14**
nearest relative, 52–3
responsible medical officer, 82
treatment, 60–61

Department of Health
circular (liability), 139
code of practice (*see* Table of Statutory Instruments)

consultation document, 6
guidance on transfers, 104
inquiry (community care), 118
memoranda, 8, 10, 15
statistics, 2, 12

Detained patients (*see also* detention), 2–3, 6
aftercare of, 115–120
and MHAC, 133–7
offences against, 139–47
transfer of, 100–104, 108

Detention, 2–3, 6, 12, 14, **15–19**, 20, **21–30**
appeals against, **72–81**, 129
date of, 100–101
information about, 49–50
in place of safety, **95–99**
mentally disordered offenders, in hospital, **33–44**
retaking/returning to, **86–91**

Disability (*see* patients with learning difficulties)

Discharge, 4, **17**, 21, 41, 43, 46, 50, **53–4**, 72–6, 78–80, 90, 108, 111, 113, **116–18**

Disposals (court orders & transfers), 36, **37–40**

Documentation, 8, **17**, **176–193**
application to MHRT, 78, 177, 183–6
faxed, 127
forgery of, 140
and guardianship, 105
and MHAC, 135, 137, 177
rectification of, **121–7**
transfers, 101, 102
treatment, 64–6

Documents (*see* documentation, records *and* Appendix II)

Duration
of court orders, 37
of guardianship order, 106
of sections, 20, 22, 24, **25**, **27–8**

ECT (electroconvulsive
therapy), 25, 26, 61, 63–4, 131
Emergency
admission, 9, 12, 20, 22, **24–6**, 30, 90, 122, 124–5
treatment, 98, 131
Errors on forms, 65, **121–4**, 131

Faxed documents, 127
Forms (see documentation, records and Appendix II), **176–193**

Guardianship, 3, 4, 9, 17, 22, 48, 50, 53, 54, 74, 76, 86, **105–109, 118**
application for, **105**
order, 36, 37–40, 43
and offences, 141–3
returning patient to, 86
transfers, 100–103

Hospital orders, 37–40

Independent medical
practitioner (see SOAD)
Informal patients, **1**, 2, 6, 8, 12, **18–22**, 27, 80, 86, 130
absence from/return to hospital, 89–90
information to, **48–9**
multidisciplinary care, 113
nearest relative, **57**
offences against, 139, 145, 146
protection of, 139, 145, **146**
transfers of, 102–103
treatment, 62, **68–9**
Information, 4, 20, **26**, 27
about detention, 49–50
checklists, 124–7
complaints procedure, 48
to detained patients, 45–51, 116, 177, 179–81
to informal patients, 48–9
to nearest relative, 45–51,

53, 85, 102, 111
to patient under section 136, 98
on treatment, 48

Judicial review, 145–6

Law Commission reports, 21, 68, 70, 175
Leave
with consent, **82–5**
without consent, **86–91**
Liability, 139–47
Living wills, 70

M'Naghten Rules, 35, 151
Mail, 133, 151
Managers, 8, 25–7, 29, 30, **129–33**
appeals to/referral by, 72–3
checklist for, 130–32
definition, 79
and documentation, 121–3, 127
duties, 17, 24, 45, 47, 78–9, 112
and MHAC, 17, 24, 45, 47, 78–9, 112
and transfers of patients, 100–104
Medical Recommendations, 7, 12, **14–18**, 20, 22, 27, 30, 36, 41, 127, 140
and admission by social worker, 112
in checklists, 124–7
and guardianship, 105
rectification of, 121
and transfers, 102
Mental Health Act
Commission (MHAC), **133–8, 178, 193**
and care of patients, 134
and documentation, 135, 137
practice notes, 62
recommendations, 118, 129
reports, 55
review of treatment, 55
Mental Health (Patients in the Community) Act 1995, 115–20, 148, 168–72
Mental Health Review
Tribunal, 17, 36, 44, 46,

49, 54, **72–81**, 148
reports to, 77
Mental incapacity, 21, 68, 175
Mentally disordered offenders (see offenders)
MHAC (see Mental Health Act Commission)
MHRT (see Mental Health Review Tribunal)
Minors, 9, 22, 53, 69
Multidisciplinary care, 113, 115

Nearest relative, 15, 20, 23, 26, 27, 44, **45–51**, **52–8**, 122
in checklists, 123–7
and guardianship, 105
and informal patient, 57
information to, 45–51
and MHRT, **72, 74**, 75, 77, 79
and social services, 102, 111, 112
Nurses
giving information, 47
holding power (section 9), 18, 20, **22–5**, **27–9**, 89–90, 97, 124, 131
implications for, **25**, 148
and mentally disordered offenders, 33, **44**
records, 66
reports, 22, 77

Offences under the act, 135, 136, **139–47**
Offenders, **33–44**, 134

Passive patients, **21**
Patient's Charter, 48, 130
Patients
informal, 1, 2, 6, 12, 18–22, 48–9, 62, 68–9
minors, 9, 22, 53, 69
passive, **21**
with learning difficulties, 9, 16, 47, 50, 60, 68
Place of safety, 40, 48, **86, 92, 96–8**
Power
doctor's holding (section 5.2), 9, 97, 123
nurse's holding (section 9.18), 20, **22–5**, **27–9**, 89–90, 97, 124, 131

Powers
  of arrest, **95–9**
  common law, 26, 29, 30, 48,
    59, 61, 90, 98
  court, **36**
  of guardian, 106, 108, 119
  Mental Health Act
    Commission, 48, 133–5
  Mental Health Review
    Tribunal, 17, 74–6
  nearest relative, 50, **43–4**
  police, 9, **95–9**
  registered medical officer,
    39, 54
  to retake patient, 87–8, 98
  Secretary of State, 35, 41, 42,
    46, 63, 133
  of social worker, 110
Prescribed medicines, 64–5
Prescribed nurse, 18, 23, **27–8,**
  29, 89, 124
Procedures (*see* code of
  practice)
Protection of staff, **143–7**

Reclassification of mental
  disorder, 17, 176
Records, 23, 26, 27, **45–7,** 49,
  51, 54, 64–6, 78, 79, 84–5,
  96
  admission, 79, 100–102, 176
  in checklists, 123–7
  correction of, **121–4**
  falsification of, 140
  inspection of, 135
  by managers, 129–30
Rectification of documents,
  121–4
Reed reports, 34
Registered
  medical practitioner, 23, 24,
    28, 38–40, 41, 54, 88, 93,
    95, 97–8, 106
  mental nursing home, 30,
    115, 129
  nurse (*see also* prescribed
    nurse), 148
Remand
  for reports, 37, 38, 40, 44
  for treatment, 37, 38, 40, 43

Renewal of section, 30–31,
  129, 176
Reports
  Audit Commission (*Finding
    a Place*), 119
  DoH (*Guidelines on
    discharge*), 118
  falsification of, 140
  from guardian, 108
  from Health Service
    Commissioner, 137
  from keyworker, 116
  to/from managers, 22, 24,
    27, 28, 67, 122
  MHAC, 55, 136–7
  for MHRT, 49
  remand for, 37, 38, 40, 44
  renewal of section, **30,** 129
  on restricted patients, 42
  by RMO, 39, 42, 46, 54, 74,
    75, 77, 79, 87
  Royal College of Psychiatrists,
    117–18
  Select Committee, 118
  from social worker, 112,
    125, 126
Responsible medical officer,
  22, 23, 25, 27, 30, 38, 41,
  42, 46, 54, **66–7,** 74, 75,
  77, 79, 87
  in checklists, 125–6
  leave/recall, 82–3, 86–7
Restraint, 20, 22, 174
Restriction direction, **42–3,** 82
Restriction order, **35, 36,** 37,
  41, 74, 76, 82
Review tribunal (*see* Mental
  Health Review Tribunal)
RMO (*see* responsible medical
  officer)

Seclusion, 67, 80, 131, 174
Second opinion approved
  doctor, 26, 36, 39, **62–4,**
  113
Secretary of State, 1, 2, 6, 129
  approved doctors (SOAD),
    15, 66
  care in the community, 119
  offenders, 35–7, 39, **41–4**

and the MHAC, 133–5
  powers, 35, 37, 39, 41–4, 46,
    57, 63, 133
  and section 57, 61
  and section 139, 146
  and treatment, 63, 67
Special hospitals, 2, 33–4, 83
SOAD (*see* second opinion
  approved doctor)
Social Services, 100–104, 105,
  112, 113, 115, 116, 117,
  120, 124, 125, 126
Social workers (*see also*
  approved social worker,
  ASW), **110–114**
Supervision order, 148
Supervision register, 119

Transfer direction, 36, 39,
  40–42
Transfers, 3, 25, 33, 35–7, 40,
  41–3, **100–104, 115, 127,**
  130, 178
Treatment, 1–3, 6, 9, 20, **22,**
  25–6, 28, 38, 39, 40, **59–71**
  application for, by social
    worker, 102, 111
  checklist for admission for,
    126–7
  in community, 115–120
  complaints about, 135–7,
    145
  consent to, 54, 59, 67, 134,
    177
  definition of, 60–61
  informal patients, 62, **68–9**
  information on, 45, 46, 48,
    49
  offenders, **43–44**
  physical disorders, 61–2
  plans, 57, 67, 113
  records, 57, 177
  remand for, 37–8, 40
  review of, 67, 133
  urgent, 62–3
  and section 17 leave, 85
  and section 136 (arrest), 98
Trusts, 8, 79, 102, 113, 129–30,
  137, 146

Section Index

Section 1, 13, 14, 24, 157

Section 2, 2, 9, 12, 16, 18, 20, 22–7, 30–2, 49, 51, 53, 54, 56, 57, 71, 73, 75, 76, 80, 87, 92, 111, 123, 126, 131, 157

Section 3, 9, 12, 18, 20, 22–26, 30, 31, 50, 51, 53, 54, 60, 62, 71, 73, 74, 76, 91, 92, 105, 109, 111, 114, 115, 123, 127, 131, 145, 146, 147, 158

Section 4, 9, 12, 16, 22–4, 26, 27, 30, 31, 50, 51, 54, 60, 74, 87, 92, 111, 112, 122, 125, 158–9

Section 5, 9, 10, 16, 18, 22–5, 27–31, 46, 50, 60, 74, 87, 89, 90, 91, 97, 100, 101, 103, 123, 124, 127, 131, 145, 159–160

Section 6, 79

Section 7, 54, 105, 106

Section 8, 106, 107

Section 11, 49, 50, 102, 105, 110, 111

Section 12, 12, 14, 15, 36, 39, 102, 122, 125, 126, 160–61

Section 13, 102, 110, 111, 112

Section 14, 112

Section 15, 12, 17, 121, 122, 132, 161

Section 16, 17, 74, 162

Section 17, 3, 9, 82–7, 91, 93, 116, 118, 146, 148, 162–3

Section 18, 9, 87, 88, 106, 107, 110, 163

Section 19, 100, 107, 108, 132

Section 20, 30, 31, 79, 87, 163

Section 21, 87

Section 23, 9, 41, 46, 50, 54, 72, 129, 130

Section 24, 54

Section 25, 46, 54, 55, 130

Section 26, 52, 53, 122

Section 29, 55, 56, 110

Section 35, 37, 38, 40, 60, 100, 103, 163

Section 36, 37, 38, 40, 43, 100, 103, 163

Section 37, 36–41, 44, 60, 74, 76, 105, 115, 163

Section 38, 37–70, 43, 74, 100, 103, 163

Section 41, 41–3, 73, 74, 83, 163

Section 42, 60

Section 47, 37, 39, 40, 42–4, 76, 115, 163

Section 48, 37, 39, 42, 43, 76, 115, 163

Section 49, 37, 42–4

Sections 50–54, 43

Section 57, 48, 61–3, 66–8, 145, 164

Section 58, 25, 26, 61–7, 85, 148, 164–5

Sections 59–60, 67

Section 61, 67, 165

Section 62, 25, 26, 61–4, 67, 131

Section 63, 25, 26, 61, 62, 67, 85, 166

Section 66, 72

Section 68, 130

Section 69, 36

Section 72, 17, 75, 76, 166

Sections 73–4, 60

Section 78, 78

Section 115, 42, 92, 93, 110

Section 117, 7, 50, 57, 112, 113, 115, 116, 119, 167

Section 118, 6

Section 120, 135

Section 121, 133, 135

Section 126, 121, 140, 141, 142

Section 127, 140–42

Section 128, 140–43

Section 129, 93, 135, 140, 142

Section 130, 140, 142

Section 131, 21, 167

Section 132, 26, 98, 130

Section 133, 50, 130

Section 135, 16, 88, 92, 93, 96, 100, 101, 110, 167

Section 136, 9, 16, 48, 60, 89, 95–101, 103, 167

Section 137, 95, 142

Section 138, 97, 110

Section 139, 139, 143–6, 167

Section 141, 143–4

Section 145, 60, 96, 129